Free Video ~~FREE~~ **Free Video**

Essential Test Tips Video from Trivium Test Prep

Dear Customer,

Thank you for purchasing from Trivium Test Prep! We're honored to help you prepare for your phlebotomy exam.

To show our appreciation, we're offering a **FREE NHA *Essential Test Tips* Video by Trivium Test Prep.*** Our video includes 35 test preparation strategies that will make you successful on your exam. All we ask is that you email us your feedback and describe your experience with our product. Amazing, awful, or just so-so: we want to hear what you have to say!

To receive your **FREE NHA *Essential Test Tips* Video**, please email us at 5star@triviumtestprep.com. Include "Free 5 Star" in the subject line and the following information in your email:

1. The title of the product you purchased.
2. Your rating from 1 – 5 (with 5 being the best).
3. Your feedback about the product, including how our materials helped you meet your goals and ways in which we can improve our products.
4. Your full name and shipping address so we can send your **FREE NHA *Essential Test Tips* Video**.

If you have any questions or concerns please feel free to contact us directly at 5star@triviumtestprep.com.

Thank you!

– Trivium Test Prep Team

*To get access to the free video please email us at 5star@triviumtestprep.com, and please follow the instructions above.

NHA PHLEBOTOMY EXAM STUDY GUIDE 2022-2023:

Test Prep Book with 400+ Practice Questions for the National Healthcareer Association Certified Phlebotomy Technician Examination [2nd Edition]

E. M. Falgout

TABLE OF CONTENTS

ONLINE RESOURCES

To help you fully prepare for your NHA Certified Phlebotomy Technician (CPT) exam, Ascencia includes online resources with the purchase of this study guide.

Practice Test

In addition to the practice test included in this book, we also offer an online exam. Since many exams today are computer based, getting to practice your test-taking skills on the computer is a great way to prepare.

Flash Cards

A convenient supplement to this study guide, Ascencia's flash cards enable you to review important terms easily on your computer or smartphone.

Cheat Sheets

Review the core skills you need to master the exam with easy-to-read Cheat Sheets.

From Stress to Success

Watch "From Stress to Success," a brief but insightful YouTube video that offers the tips, tricks, and secrets experts use to score higher on the exam.

Reviews

Leave a review, send us helpful feedback, or sign up for Ascencia promotions—including free books!

Access these materials at: **www.ascenciatestprep.com/nha-phlebotomy-online-resources**

INTRODUCTION

Congratulations on choosing to take the NHA Certified Phlebotomy Technician (CPT) exam! Passing the CPT exam is an important step forward in your health care career. In the following pages, you will find information about the exam, what to expect on test day, how to use this book, and the content covered on the exam.

The Certification Process

The **National Healthcareer Association (NHA)** is a professional organization that offers certifications for medical assistants and technicians. Their **Phlebotomy Technician Certification (CPT)** exam is offered as part of their process for becoming a certified phlebotomy technician.

To qualify for the CPT exam, you must have a combination of academic and professional experience that includes:

- high school graduation or equivalent;
- the successful completion of a qualifying training program within the last five years OR at least one year of supervised work experience in the health field covered by the NHA certification exam within the last three years;
- documented performance of a minimum of thirty (30) venipunctures and ten (10) capillary sticks on live individuals.

Once you have passed the exam, your certification will last for two years, and you may use the credentials as long as your certification is valid. After this period, you will need to recertify by fulfilling continuing education requirements.

Questions and Timing

During the CPT exam you'll have **two hours** to answer **120 questions**. Only one hundred of these questions are scored; twenty are unscored, or *pretest* questions. These questions are included by the NHA to test their suitability for inclusion in future tests. You'll have no way of knowing which questions are unscored, so treat every question like it counts.

The questions on the phlebotomy technician exam are multiple choice with four answer options. The exam has **no guess penalty**. That is, if you answer a question incorrectly, no points are deducted from your score; you simply do not get credit for that question. Therefore, you should always guess if you do not know the answer to a question.

Content Areas

The content of the CPT exam covers the concepts and skills necessary for success as a phlebotomist. Questions will cover both tasks and theoretical knowledge. The test plan describes five content areas covered on the NHA CPT exam.

Plan for the NHA CPT Exam

Content Area	Description
Safety and Compliance	Workplace safety, operational standards, scope of practice, ethics, quality control, infection control
Patient Preparation	Patient identification, consent, requisition forms, special considerations for collections, testing requirements, patient interview techniques
Routine Blood Collections	Equipment, techniques, and procedures for venipuncture
Special Collections	Equipment, techniques, and procedures for blood smears; blood cultures, non-blood specimens
Processing	Preparing, transporting, and processing specimens; point-of-care testing

Exam Administration

To register for the exam, you must first apply through the NHA (https://www.nhanow.com). You will be asked to submit the necessary documents to demonstrate that you meet the eligibility requirements.

When registering for the exam, you will be asked to choose a test location. The CPT exam may be taken through an affiliated school, employer, or at a PSI testing center. If you choose to take the exam at an affiliated institution, you will need to select a specific test date. If you need to use a PSI testing center, you will need to register for an available date on the PSI website (https://candidate.psiexams.com).

On the day of the exam, be prepared to bring at least one form of **government-issued photo ID** that includes a current photograph, your signature, and a permanent address. If you do not have proper ID, you will not be allowed to take the test.

In most locations, the test will be given on a computer. You will have the opportunity to take a short tutorial before the exam begins to familiarize yourself with the testing software. Some sites will offer a pencil-and-paper exam; you will need to bring No. 2 pencils if you are taking the test on paper.

Exam Results

The NHA will email you a notification when your test results are available, and you may view your score through the candidate portal. Your raw score is how many of the one hundred scored questions you answer correctly. That score is then scaled from 200 to 500 based on the level of difficulty of the questions you answer correctly. The phlebotomy technician exam is a pass/fail test. The minimum passing scaled score is 390. Your score report will provide your scaled score and a status of pass or fail.

If you do not pass the exam, you may retake it after a thirty-day waiting period. You will have three opportunities to take the exam; if none of these are successful, you will need to wait one year before you can reapply to take the exam again.

Using This Book

This book is divided into two sections. In the content area review, you will find a review of the knowledge and skills included in the exam content outline. Throughout the chapter you'll also see Quick Review Questions that will help reinforce important concepts and skills.

The book also includes two full-length practice tests (one in the book and one online) with answer rationales. You can use these tests to gauge your readiness for the exam and determine which content areas you may need to review more thoroughly.

Ascencia Test Prep

With health care fields such as nursing, pharmacy, emergency care, and physical therapy becoming the fastest-growing industries in the United States, individuals looking to enter the health care industry or rise in their field need high-quality, reliable resources. Ascencia Test Prep's study guides and test preparation materials are developed by credentialed industry professionals with years of experience in their respective fields. Ascencia recognizes that health care professionals nurture bodies and spirits, and save lives. Ascencia Test Prep's mission is to help health care workers grow.

ONE: ANATOMY and PHYSIOLOGY

The Biological Hierarchy

- The biological hierarchy is a systematic classification of the structures of the human body, from smallest to largest (or largest to smallest).

- The smallest unit of the human body is the **cell**, a microscopic, self-replicating structure. Different types of cells have different functions.

- **Tissues** are the next largest group of structures in the body. Each tissue is a collection of cells that perform a similar function. The human body has four basic types of tissues:
  - **Connective** tissues—which include bones, ligaments, and cartilage— *meninges* support, separate, or connect the body's various organs and other tissues.
  - **Epithelial** tissues are found in the skin, blood vessels, and many organs.
  - **Muscular** tissues contain contractile units that pull on connective tissues to create movement.
  - **Nervous** tissue makes up the peripheral nervous system, which transmits impulses throughout the body.

- **Organs** are collections of tissues within the body that perform a certain function (e.g., the esophagus or heart).

- **Organ systems** are a group of organs that work together to perform related functions (e.g., the digestive system).

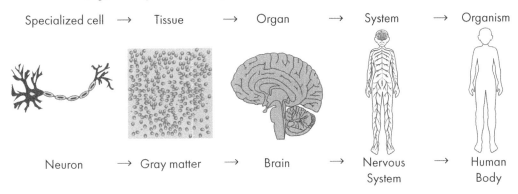

Specialized cell → Tissue → Organ → System → Organism

Neuron → Gray matter → Brain → Nervous System → Human Body

Figure 1.1. Biological Hierarchy and Levels of Organization

- Finally, an **organism** is the total collection of all the parts of the biological hierarchy working together to form a living being. It is the largest structure in the biological hierarchy.

QUICK REVIEW QUESTION

1. The meninges are membranes that surround and protect the brain and spinal cord. What type of tissue are the meninges? *Connective tissue*

Directional Terminology and Planes

- When discussing anatomy and physiology, specific terms are used to refer to directions (in anatomy, the terms "right" and "left" are used with respect to the subject, not the observer).

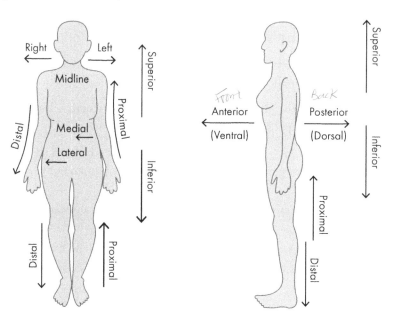

Figure 1.2. Directional Terms

- Directional terms include:
  - **inferior**: away from the head
  - **superior**: closer to the head
  - **anterior**: toward the front
  - **posterior**: toward the back
  - **dorsal**: toward the back
  - **ventral**: toward the front
  - **medial**: toward the midline of the body
  - **lateral**: away from the midline of the body
  - **proximal**: closer to the trunk
  - **distal**: away from the trunk
- The human body is divided by three imaginary planes:

- The **transverse plane** divides the body into top and bottom halves.
- The **frontal (or coronal) plane** divides the body into front and back halves.
- The **sagittal plane** divides the body into right and left halves.

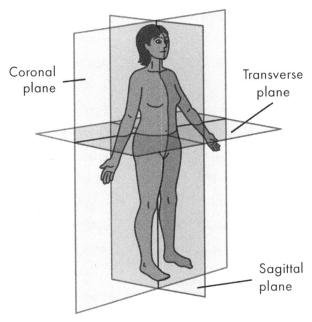

Coronal plane

Transverse plane

Sagittal plane

Figure 1.3. Planes of the Human Body

Neck is inferior to the head

QUICK REVIEW QUESTION

2. Which directional term describes the position of the neck relative to the head?

Body Systems

- The **cardiovascular system** carries oxygen, nutrients, and waste products to and from all the cells of the body via the blood. (The cardiovascular system is discussed in detail below.)
- The lymphatic system circulates **lymph**, a fluid composed of interstitial fluid and other elements.
    - Lymph flows through lymphatic vessels and **lymph nodes**, which filter out pathogens.
    - The main purpose of the lymphatic system is to return interstitial fluid to the circulatory system.
    - The lymphatic system also circulates white blood cells and fats from the digestive system.
- The **respiratory system** takes in oxygen (which is needed for cellular functioning) and expels carbon dioxide.
    - Humans take in air primarily through the nose, but also through the mouth.
    - Air travels down the **trachea** and **bronchi** into the **lungs**.
    - The lungs contain millions of small **alveoli** where oxygen and carbon dioxide are exchanged between the blood and the air.

DID YOU KNOW?
Intracellular fluid (ICF) is the fluid found inside cells. **Extracellular fluid (ECF)** is fluid in the body outside the cells. ECF includes blood plasma and interstitial fluid (the fluid that surrounds cells). Around one-third of the fluid in the body is ECF.

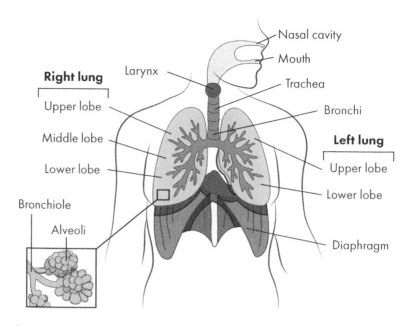

Figure 1.4. Respiratory Tract

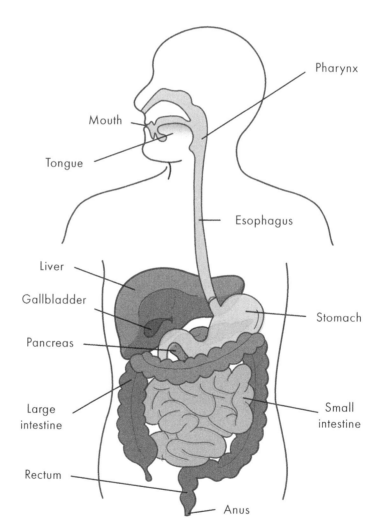

Figure 1.5. The Digestive System

- The **digestive system** breaks food down into nutrients for use by the body's cells.
  - Food enters through the **mouth** and moves through the **esophagus** to the **stomach**, where it is physically and chemically broken down.
  - The food particles then move into the **small intestine**, where the majority of nutrients are absorbed.
  - Finally, the remaining particles enter the **large intestine**, which absorbs water, and waste exits through the **rectum** and **anus**.
  - This system also include other organs, including the **liver**, **gallbladder**, and **pancreas**, that manufacture substances needed for digestion.
- The **urinary system** removes waste products from the body.
  - The **kidneys** filter waste from the bloodstream to create **urine**.
  - Urine is stored in the **bladder** and excreted via the **urethra**.

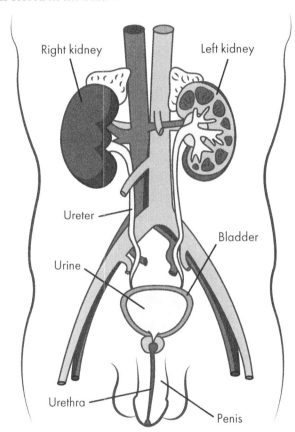

Figure 1.6. The Urinary System

- The **skeletal system** is composed of the body's **bones** and **joints**.
  - Bones and joints provide support for the body and contribute to movement.
  - Bones also store some of the body's nutrients and produce red and white blood cells.
- The **muscular system** allows the body to move and moves blood and other substances through the body.
  - **Skeletal muscles** are voluntary muscles (meaning they can be controlled) that are attached to bones and move the body.

- o **Smooth muscles** are involuntary muscles (meaning they cannot be controlled) that create movement in parts of the digestive tract, blood vessels, and reproductive system.
  - o **Cardiac muscle** is the involuntary muscle that contracts the heart, allowing it to pump blood throughout the body.
- The **immune system** protects the body from infection caused by foreign particles and organisms.
  - o It includes the **skin** and mucous membranes, which act as physical barriers.
  - o The immune system also includes specialized white blood cells that destroy foreign substances in the body.
  - o The human body has an **adaptive immune system**, meaning it can recognize and respond to foreign substances once it has been exposed to them.
- The **nervous system** processes external stimuli and sends signals throughout the body.
  - o The **central nervous system (CNS)** consists of the brain and spinal cord. It is where information is processed and stored.
  - o The **peripheral nervous system (PNS)** includes small cells called neurons that transmit information throughout the body using electrical signals.
- The **endocrine system** is a collection of **glands** that produce **hormones**, which are chemicals that regulate bodily processes.
  - o The **pancreas** produces insulin and glucagon, which regulate blood glucose levels.
  - o The **thyroid gland** produces hormones that regulate the body's metabolism.
  - o The **pituitary gland** produces hormones that control growth and regulate other glands.
  - o The **adrenal glands** produce cortisol and epinephrine, hormones that help the body regulate stress and its response to danger.
- The **reproductive system** includes the organs necessary for sexual reproduction.
  - o In males, these include the **testes**, where sperm is produced, and the **urethra**, which carries sperm through the **penis**.
  - o The female reproductive system includes the **ovaries**, where eggs are produced, and the **uterus**, where fertilized eggs develop.

QUICK REVIEW QUESTIONS

3. What is the primary function of the respiratory system?

4. What are some commonly ordered diagnostic tests related to endocrine system functioning?

The Heart

- The **heart** is a muscular organ that pumps blood throughout the body.
- The circulatory system is a closed double loop.

- In the **pulmonary loop**, deoxygenated blood leaves the heart and travels to the lungs, where it loses carbon dioxide and receives oxygen. The oxygenated blood then returns to the heart.
- The heart then pumps blood through the **systemic loop**, which delivers oxygenated blood to the rest of the body and returns deoxygenated blood to the heart.

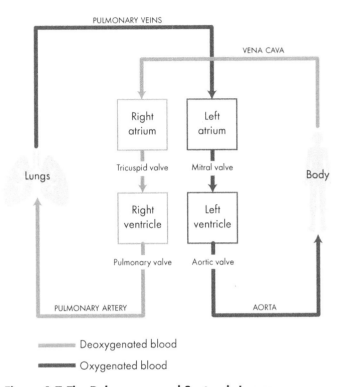

Figure 1.7. The Pulmonary and Systemic Loops

- The **heart** has four chambers:
  - The **right atrium** collects blood from the body.
  - The **right ventricle** pumps blood to the lungs.
  - The **left atrium** collects blood from the lungs.
  - The **left ventricle** pumps blood to the body.
- The **atrioventricular valves** are located between the atria and ventricles:
  - The **tricuspid valve** separates the right atrium and right ventricle.
  - The **mitral valve** separates the left atrium and left ventricle.
- The two **semilunar valves** are located between the ventricles and arteries:
  - The **pulmonary valve** separates the right ventricle and pulmonary artery.
  - The **aortic valve** separates the left ventricle and aorta.
- The heart includes several layers of tissue:
  - **pericardium**: the outermost protective layer of the heart, which contains a lubricating liquid
  - **epicardium**: the deepest layer of the pericardium, which envelops the heart muscle

○ **myocardium:** the heart muscle

○ **endocardium:** the innermost, smooth layer of the heart walls

- The heart's pumping action is regulated by the **cardiac conduction system**, which produces and conducts electrical signals in the heart:

   ○ The **sinoatrial (SA) node** sets the heart's pace by sending out electrical signals that cause the atria to contract.

   ○ The **atrioventricular (AV) node** relays the electrical impulse of the sinoatrial node to the ventricles. The impulse is delayed to allow the atria to fully contract and fill the ventricles.

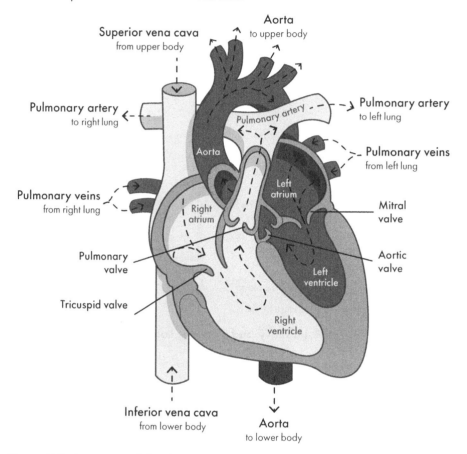

Figure 1.8. Anatomy of the Heart

QUICK REVIEW QUESTION

5.   Left-sided heart failure can cause pulmonary edema (fluid in the lungs), while right-sided heart failure is more likely to cause edema in the abdomen and extremities. How does the anatomy of the heart produce this difference?

Structure of Blood

- The cardiovascular system circulates **blood**, which carries nutrients, waste products, hormones, and other important substances throughout the body.

- **Plasma** (also called blood plasma) is the liquid part of the blood.

- Plasma is a yellow fluid composed mostly of water.
- Elements suspended or dissolved in the plasma include gases, electrolytes, carbohydrates, fats, proteins, clotting factors, and waste products.

- The cells suspended in plasma are the **formed elements**.
  - **Red blood cells (RBCs)** transport oxygen throughout the body. RBCs contain **hemoglobin**, a large molecule with iron atoms that bind to oxygen.
  - **White blood cells (WBCs)** fight infection.
  - **Platelets** (also called thrombocytes) gather at sites of damage in blood vessels as part of the blood-clotting process.

- To collect plasma, the blood specimen must be treated with an anticoagulant.
  - Blood specimens with an added anticoagulant are called **whole-blood specimens**.
  - When centrifuged, whole-blood specimens will separate into three layers: plasma, white blood cells and platelets (**buffy coat**), and red blood cells.

- **Serum** is plasma with clotting factors (fibrinogen) removed.
  - Serum is collected by allowing a blood specimen to coagulate.
  - After centrifugation, a serum tube will have two layers: serum and clotted blood.
  - In a serum separator tube (SST), a gel layer will separate the serum from the clotted blood.

Plasma specimen
(with anticoagulant)

Serum specimen
(without anticoagulant)

Serum specimen
with separating gel

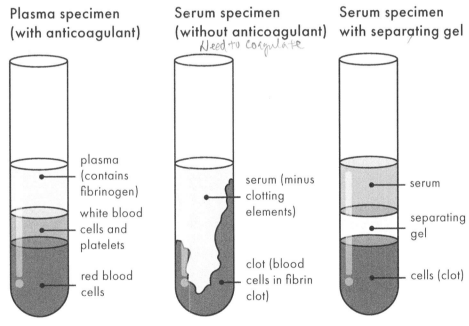

Figure 1.9. Centrifuged Blood Specimens

- **Blood groups** (also called blood types) are determined by the presence of **antigens**, proteins that activate antibodies.
  - **Antibodies** are immune system proteins that bind to antigens to destroy the attached cell or pathogen.

- Each blood group produces specific antibodies that attach to antigens on RBCs.
- When antibodies attack RBCs, the cells will **agglutinate** (clump) and **lyse** (break apart), a process called a **transfusion reaction**.
- When receiving a blood transfusion, a person should receive their own blood type to avoid a transfusion reaction.

- The **ABO blood group** is defined by the presence or absence of A antigens and B antigens.
  - A person's RBC may contain A antigens, B antigens, both antigens, or neither antigen.
  - If a person does not have one type of antigen, their plasma will contain antibodies that attack that antigen (e.g., a person with type A blood will have antibodies that attack type B blood cells).

Table 1.1. The ABO Blood Groups

Blood Type	Antigens on RBC	Antibodies in Plasma
A	A antigens	anti-B antibodies
B	B antigens	anti-A antibodies
O	no antigens	anti-A and anti-B antibodies
AB	A and B antigens	no antibodies

- The Rh blood group is defined by the presence of **Rh factor**, an antigen also called the D antigen.
  - The blood type **Rh-positive** has Rh factor antigens on RBCs.
  - The blood type **Rh-negative** does not have Rh factor antigens on RBCs.
  - Anti-Rh antibodies develop when Rh-negative blood is exposed to Rh factor.
  - In **hemolytic disease of the newborn**, anti-Rh antibodies in an Rh-negative mother attack the RBCs of her Rh-positive fetus.

QUICK REVIEW QUESTIONS

6. What function do red blood cells perform in the human body?

7. Why is an anticoagulant needed to collect a plasma sample for diagnostic testing?

The Coagulation Process

- **Hemostasis** is the process of stopping blood loss from a damaged blood vessel.
- Blood loss is stopped through **coagulation**, the process of turning liquid blood into a semisolid clot.
- A **clot** is composed of platelets and red blood cells held together by the protein **fibrin**.
- The hemostatic process involves four steps:
  - vasoconstriction, the narrowing of the blood vessels that slows blood flow to the injured area

- formation of a **platelet plug** (or **hemostatic plug**), a temporary mass formed when platelets stick to each other during **platelet aggregation**
- formation of a **secondary plug** with fibrin, which is longer-lasting and more stable
- **fibrinolysis**, the disintegration of the blood clot
- The process of coagulation is a complex cascade of reactions involving proteins called **clotting factors**.
  - Platelet aggregation is initiated by the exposure to **von Willebrand factor (vW)** and **tissue factor (TF)**.
  - During coagulation, the protein **fibrinogen** (factor I) is converted to fibrin by the enzyme **thrombin** (factor IIa).
  - **Prothrombin** (factor II) is a precursor to thrombin.
  - **Hemophilia** is caused by a deficiency of factor VIII or factor IX.

QUICK REVIEW QUESTION

8. Von Willebrand disease is caused by low levels or poor quality of von Willebrand factor. What signs and symptoms would a patient with von Willebrand disease likely have? *excessive bleeding   or Anemia*

Blood Vessels

- Blood leaves the heart and travels throughout the body in **blood vessels**, which decrease in diameter as they move away from the heart and toward the tissues and organs.

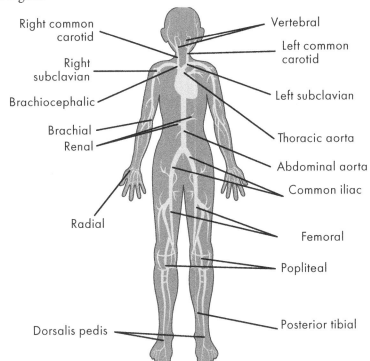

Figure 1.10. Major Arteries

- Blood exits the heart through **arteries**.

- The arteries branch into **arterioles** and then **capillaries**, where gas exchange between blood and tissue takes place.

- **Venules** are small veins that collect deoxygenated blood from capillaries.

- Venules feed into larger **veins**, which return blood to the heart.

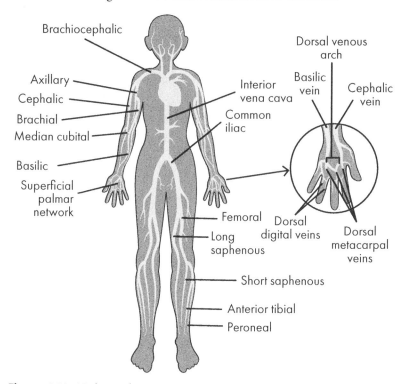

Figure 1.11. Major Veins

- Some veins have **valves** that prevent deoxygenated blood from flowing back to the extremities.

- Blood vessels have three layers:
  ○ the **tunica adventitia**, the outer layer, composed of connective tissue
  ○ the **tunica media**, the middle layer, composed of smooth muscle
  ○ the **tunica intima**, the thin inner layer

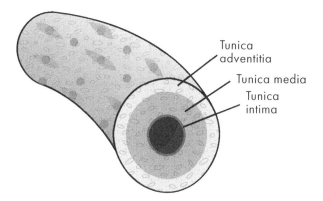

Figure 1.12. Structure of Blood Vessels

- The **lumen** is the interior space of the blood vessel, through which blood flows.

QUICK REVIEW QUESTION

9.   Describe the pathway that oxygenated blood takes after it leaves the heart and travels through the different types of blood vessels.

Assessing Cardiovascular Function

- The heart beats a certain number of times each minute, a value called the **pulse**, or **heart rate**.
  - ○ The pulse can be taken at a number of locations on the body:
    - · radial pulse, on the thumb side of the inner wrist (most commonly used)
    - · carotid pulse, to the side of the trachea
    - · brachial pulse, on the side of crease of the elbow
  - ○ The pulse is measured as the number of times the heart beats in 1 minute.
  - ○ The average adult's pulse rate at rest is between 60 and 100 beats per minute.
- **Blood pressure (BP)** is the measurement of the force of blood as it flows against the walls of the arteries, measured in mm Hg.
  - ○ **Systolic pressure** is the pressure that occurs while the heart is contracting.
  - ○ **Diastolic pressure** occurs while the heart is relaxed.
  - ○ A healthy blood pressure has a systolic value of 100 to 139 mm Hg and a diastolic value of 60 to 79 mm Hg.
- An **electrocardiogram (ECG)** is a noninvasive diagnostic tool that records the heart's electrical activity.
  - ○ ECGs help determine a patient's cardiac rhythm and rate and can also help diagnose electrolyte imbalances, heart attacks, and other damage to the heart.
  - ○ The readout from the ECG, often called an ECG strip, is a continuous waveform whose shape corresponds to each stage in the cardiac cycle:
    - · **P wave**: right and left atrial contraction and depolarization
    - · **QRS complex**: contraction of the ventricles
    - · **T wave**: relaxation of the ventricles and repolarization
  - ○ A normal heart rhythm and rate is called normal sinus rhythm.

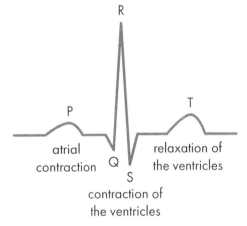

Figure 1.13. Waveforms and Intervals on ECG

QUICK REVIEW QUESTION

10. If a rhythm is missing P waves or has an excessive number of P waves, which area of the heart is having difficulty conducting?

Answer Key

1. The meninges are connective tissue.

2. The neck is inferior to, or below, the head.

3. The primary function of the respiratory system is the intake of oxygen and the exhalation of carbon dioxide.

4. Glucose tolerance tests are used to test for disorders related to insulin production; insulin and glucagon levels can also be directly measured. Common tests for hormone levels include thyroid function tests and tests for human growth hormone, cortisol, and antidiuretic hormone (which regulates urine production).

5. Blood from the lungs is returned to the left side of the heart. When the left side cannot pump this blood back out to the body, fluid builds up in the lungs. Blood from the body is returned to the right side of the heart, so right-sided failure causes fluid to build up in the abdomen and extremities.

6. Red blood cells (RBCs) carry oxygen throughout the body so it can be absorbed into cells and used for cellular respiration. Oxygen is carried on hemoglobin, an iron-containing protein found in RBCs.

7. Plasma is the liquid portion of the blood, which includes clotting factors (fibrinogen). When blood is allowed to clot naturally, the clotting factors are trapped in the blood clot, leaving serum behind. To collect a plasma sample, the blood must be prevented from clotting so that clotting factors remain in the specimen. The sample can then be centrifuged to separate the plasma from the RBCs.

8. People with von Willebrand disease will bleed easily and for longer periods of time. Symptoms range from easy bruising and nosebleeds to life-threatening hemorrhages following trauma or surgery.

9. Oxygenated blood leaves the heart from the left ventricle. It travels through the aorta, the largest artery in the body. The blood then travels through arteries until it reaches smaller vessels: the arterioles and then capillaries. Gas exchange takes place in the capillaries. The deoxygenated blood is collected from capillaries into venules and then into veins, which carry the blood back to the heart.

10. The P wave shows atrial depolarization. If a rhythm shows abnormalities in the P waves, then the patient's atria are not functioning properly.

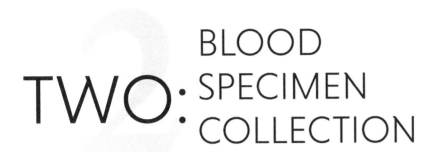

TWO: BLOOD SPECIMEN COLLECTION

Venipuncture Equipment

- Vein puncture or **venipuncture** is the puncturing of the skin to collect blood from a vein. Blood can be collected:
  - for diagnostic testing
  - for donation
  - as medical therapy

Table 2.1. Common Diagnostic Blood Tests

Test Name	Tests For ...
Complete Blood Count (CBC)	
White blood cells (WBCs)	number of WBCs in blood; increased number of WBCs can indicate inflammation or infection
Red blood cells (RBCs)	number of RBCs, which carry oxygen throughout the body and filter carbon dioxide
Hemoglobin (HgB)	amount of hemoglobin, a protein that holds oxygen in the blood
Hematocrit (Hct)	percentage of the blood composed of red blood cells
Mean corpuscular volume (MCV)	average size of red blood cells
Mean corpuscular hemoglobin (MCH)	average amount of hemoglobin per RBC
Mean corpuscular hemoglobin concentration (MCHC)	average concentration of hemoglobin in RBCs
Platelets	number of platelets, which play a role in the body's clotting process

Table 2.1. Common Diagnostic Blood Tests (continued)

Test Name	Tests For ...
Coagulation Tests	
Prothrombin time (PT)	how long it takes blood to clot
International normalized ratio (INR)	effectiveness of an anticoagulant in thinning blood
Partial thromboplastin time (PTT)	the body's ability to form blood clots
Activated partial thromboplastin time (aPTT)	the body's ability to form blood clots using an activator to speed up the clotting process
D-dimer	protein fragments left in the blood when clots dissolve
Fibrinogen	levels of fibrinogen, a protein necessary for clotting
Thrombin time	function of thrombin, an enzyme that acts on fibrinogen during the clotting process
Chemistry Panels	
Kidney function tests	components related to kidney function (e.g., electrolytes, blood urea nitrogen [BUN], and creatinine)
Liver function tests	components related to liver function (e.g., bilirubin levels, ALT, AST)
Basic metabolic panel (BMP)	components related to metabolism (e.g., glucose) and kidney function
Comprehensive metabolic panel (CMP)	BMP plus proteins and liver function
Lipid profile	fats in the blood, including cholesterol, low-density lipoprotein (LDL), and high-density lipoprotein (HDL)
Other Serology and Immunology Tests	
Tests for specific infections	antibodies for various bacterial and viral infections, including HIV, cytomegalovirus, Epstein-Barr, hepatitis, and syphilis
Cold agglutinins	antibodies that attack RBCs; may be autoimmune or triggered by infection
C-reactive protein (CRP)	a protein produced in the liver; found in increased amounts when inflammation is present
Erythrocyte sedimentation rate (ESR)	rate of RBC sedimentation, which is affected by proteins caused by inflammation
Pregnancy test	human chorionic gonadotropin (hCG), a hormone produced by the placenta

- Venipuncture can be done using one of three different systems:
  - evacuated tube system (most common)

- syringe system (used for difficult collections)
- winged infusion blood collection set; also called a butterfly (used for small veins, usually in pediatric and elderly patients)

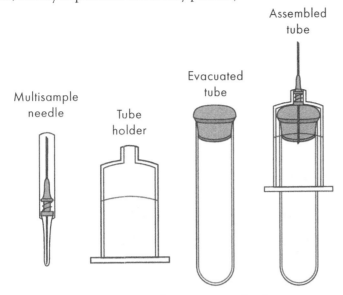

Figure 2.1. Components of an Evacuated Tube System

- Venipuncture needles come in several varieties and sizes including **multi-sample needles** (for ETS), **hypodermic** needles (for syringe system), and **winged** or **butterfly needles**.
  - The **gauge** of a needle refers to the **lumen diameter** of the needle and is selected based on the size and condition of the patient's vein. The higher the gauge, the smaller the diameter of the needle.
  - Some common types of needles and their uses are below:
    - 15- to 17-gauge: donor unit collection or therapeutic phlebotomy
    - 20-gauge multi-sample: large volume tubes, for adults with normal-sized veins
    - 21-gauge multi-sample: standard venipuncture needle for patients with normal-sized veins
    - 22-gauge multi-sample syringe: for older children or adults with small or "difficult" veins   *ABG*
    - 23-gauge butterfly: for infants and children and hand veins of adults
    - 25-gauge butterfly: for premature/neonate scalp veins
- An **evacuated tube system (ETS)** is a closed system that draws blood directly from the vein and allows for a multi-sample collection from one vein puncture.
  - An ETS has three components: evacuated tubes, a tube holder, and a multi-sample venipuncture needle.
  - Multiple tubes can be filled in succession by removing one from the tube holder and placing another one once the needle has been placed in a vein.
- **Evacuated tubes** draw a predetermined amount of blood directly into the tube.
  - When evacuated tubes are made, air is removed from the tube to create a vacuum.

HELPFUL HINT

Do not disconnect the tube holder from the needle after blood draw. Place the entire unit (tube holder and needle) into the sharps container.

- ○ When the tube is placed in the tube holder, blood from the vein will fill the vacuum in the tube.
- ○ Tube labels list the recommended **fill volume**. Filling the tube until the vacuum is exhausted will ensure the correct amount of blood is collected.
- ○ **Expiration dates** are printed on each evacuated tube. Expired tubes should not be used because they may not fill completely (due to ineffective vacuum).
- ○ The color of the tube cap indicates which additive is included.
- **Additives** are included in evacuated tubes to help preserve specimens or prepare them for testing.
  - ○ **Anticoagulants** prevent blood from clotting.
  - ○ **Clot activators** accelerate the clotting process.
  - ○ **Antiglycolytics** prevent glycolysis (breakdown of blood glucose by blood cells).
  - ○ **Dextrose** nourishes and preserves cells.
  - ○ **Gel separators** provide a physical barrier between cells and serum or plasma when the tube is centrifuged.
- During a multi-sample collection, tubes need to be collected in a specific **order of draw** to prevent additive cross contamination between tubes.
  - ○ Order of draw is established by the Clinical and Laboratory Standards Institute (CLSI).
  - ○ If a tube is drawn out of order, draw another tube and discard the original. If more tubes need to be collected, draw a discard tube before continuing.

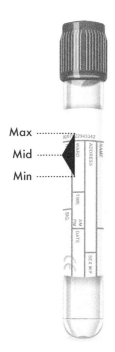

Max ....
Mid ....
Min ....

Figure 2.2. Recommended Fill Lines on Evacuated Tube

Table 2.2. Evacuated Tube Additives and Order of Draw

Order of Draw	Type of Collection	Commonly Used For . . .	Color	Additive	Number of Inversions
1	blood cultures	blood cultures	yellow	**sodium polyanethol sulfonate (SPS)**, an anticoagulant that reduces damage to bacteria	8
2	sodium citrate tubes	coagulation tests	light blue	**sodium citrate**, an anticoagulant	3 – 4
3	serum tubes	chemistry tests (e.g., metabolic panel, lipid panel)	red	**silica**, a clot activator	5 – 10
			red and gray; gold	**serum separator tube (SST)** with silica and separator gel	5 – 10
			orange	**rapid serum tube (RST) with thrombin**, a fast-acting anticoagulant	5 – 10

Order of Draw	Type of Collection	Commonly Used For . . .	Color	Additive	Number of Inversions
4	heparin tubes	stat chemistry tests	dark green	**heparin**, an anti-coagulant	5 – 10
			light green; green and gray	**plasma separator tube (PST)** with heparin and gel separator	5 – 10
5	EDTA tubes	hematology tests (e.g., CBC, blood bank testing)	lavender; pink	**EDTA**, an antico-agulant	8 – 10
			pearl/ white	**plasma prepa-ration tube (PPT)** with EDTA and gel separator	8 – 10
6	sodium fluoride or potassium oxalate	glucose tests, ethanol test	gray	**sodium fluoride**, an antiglyco-lytic agent, or **potassium oxalate**, an anti-coagulant	8 – 10
7	acid citrate dextrose (ACD)	DNA testing, transplant compatibility	yellow	**acid citrate dextrose (ACD)**, an anticoagulant (acid citrate) and RBC preservative (dextrose)	8
N/A	trace-element-free tubes	toxicology, trace element tests	royal blue	free of trace element contam-ination and may contain other additives (drawn in order of additives)	varies

HELPFUL HINT

Below is a simplified order of draw:

cultures	yellow
citrate	light blue
serum	red/orange
heparin	green
EDTA	lavender/pink
fluoride	gray

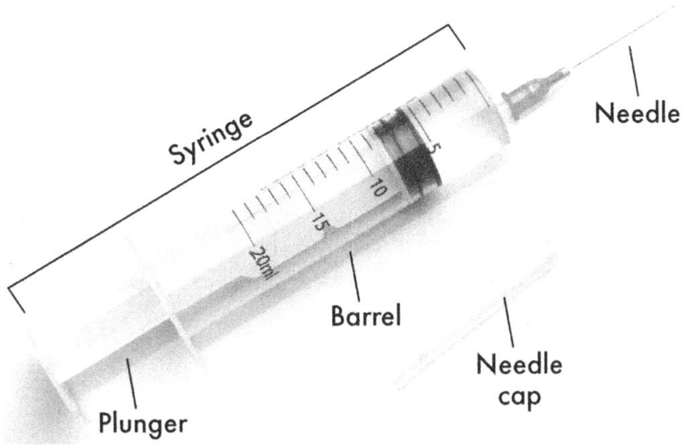

Figure 2.3. Parts of a Syringe

- A **syringe system** consists of a hypodermic needle and syringe with a Luer lock.
  - The **syringe** has a cylindrical **barrel** and a **plunger**, which is a rod-like device within the barrel that is gently pulled back to fill the syringe with blood.
  - **Syringe needles** are usually 21 – 23 gauge, 1 – 1.5 inches (2.5 – 3.8 cm) long, and have an attached re-sheathing device to decrease the risk of an accidental needlestick.
  - Blood collected in a syringe is transferred to an ETS tube using a **syringe transfer device** that is placed on the syringe after the needle has been removed.
  - When filling tubes, the phlebotomist must hold syringe transfer devices vertically pointing downward to prevent contamination.

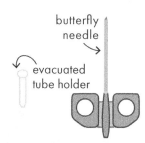

butterfly needle

evacuated tube holder

tubing

Figure 2.5. Winged Infusion Set Attached to an Evacuated Tube Holder

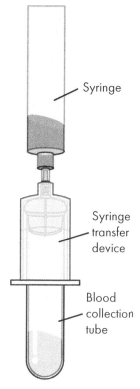

Syringe

Syringe transfer device

Blood collection tube

Figure 2.4. Syringe Transfer Device

- A **winged infusion** blood collection set (or **butterfly**) consists of a 0.5 – 0.75 inch (1.3 – 1.9 cm) needle with plastic extension "wings" connected to a 5 – 12 inch (12.7 – 30.5 cm) tubing.
  - The tubing can be attached to a syringe or an evacuated tube holder.
  - Smaller needle sizes should be used with caution since they can cause hemolysis.
  - The first draw from a butterfly should be discarded because air in the tubing will cause the first evacuated tube to be underfilled.

- **Tourniquets** and **vein viewers** can be used when veins are difficult to identify or locate.

- **Tourniquets** are elastic bands wrapped around the arm that restrict the flow of blood through veins out of the arm, causing the veins to expand and making them easier to puncture.
  - A tourniquet should not be used for more than 1 minute since this can change the blood components.
  - Bands may be single-use (disposable) or multiuse (non-disposable).
  - Multiuse tourniquets should be disinfected often.
  - If a plastic band is not available, a manual blood pressure cuff can be inflated.

- **Vein viewers** are vein-locating devices that use transillumination to identify veins under the skin. Light is projected onto the skin, and hemoglobin in the blood absorbs the light, making veins appear darker than surrounding tissue.

DID YOU KNOW?

A *discard tube* is an evacuated tube with no additive or the same additive as the first draw that is filled and discarded. It is used when the first draw is likely contaminated or damaged (e.g., with a heplock or a butterfly).

QUICK REVIEW QUESTIONS

1. What size needle would be most commonly selected for each of the following situations?

a) 19-year-old healthy patient donating blood

b) hand vein on 60-year-old patient

c) premature infant in the NICU

d) 30-year-old healthy patient having routine lab work

2. A phlebotomist needs to draw a PPT, an SST, and a citrate tube. In what order should the tubes be drawn?

3. A provider suspects that a patient has anemia (a decreased number of RBCs). Which test will the provider order to confirm the diagnosis? What type of evacuated tube would be used to collect this specimen?

Safety and Infection Control Equipment

- The **patient chair** often has a reclining feature or locking armrest to prevent a patient from falling.

- Supplies are stored in a portable carrier or a cart.
  - A **portable carrier** can be used in emergent situations or when a patient cannot easily move to the phlebotomy chair.
  - A **supply cart** stores equipment for a large number of specimen collections.

- **Infection control supplies** play an important role in maintaining a clean, safe environment for patients and staff.

- **Antiseptics** prevent the growth of microorganisms on the skin.
  - Antiseptics are used to clean skin at the venipuncture site prior to blood draw.
  - **70% isopropyl alcohol** is the most common antiseptic.
  - Other antiseptics include 70% ethyl alcohol, benzalkonium chloride, chlorhexidine gluconate, hydrogen peroxide, tincture of iodine, and povidone-iodine swabs.

- **Disinfectants** remove or kill microorganisms on instruments and work surfaces.
  - Disinfectants are not safe for use on human skin.
  - **Sodium hypochlorite** (bleach) is the most common disinfectant.

- The Occupational Safety and Health Administration (OSHA) requires that **gloves** be used during venipuncture.
  - Gloves must be changed between each patient.
  - Gloves should be latex-free to avoid causing an allergic reaction in patients.

- Alcohol-based **hand sanitizer** is acceptable for routine hand hygiene.
  - If hands are visibly soiled, hand sanitizer alone is not sufficient.

- Needle safety precautions include:
  - Dispose of all needles, lancets, and sharps in a **sharps container**.
  - All needle and puncture devices must be sealed in sterile, one-time use containers.
  - If a seal is broken, dispose of the equipment in a sharps container.
  - Inspect all needles for manufacturing defects such as barbs and blunt tips.

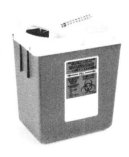

Figure 2.6. Sharps Container

HELPFUL HINT

Do not overfill a sharps container or attempt to forcefully push additional needles into the container. This can result in an accidental needlestick.

4. What is the difference between an antiseptic and a disinfectant? When should each one be used by a phlebotomist?

Preparing the Patient

1. Begin by reviewing and clarifying orders on the requisition form, which lists the tests the patient's provider would like to have drawn. (See chapter 4 for more detailed information on requisition forms.)
   - ○ Verify that all required information is present and complete.
   - ○ Confirm which tests are being collected as well as date and time of collection.
   - ○ Review diet restrictions needed prior to collection.
   - ○ Check test status priority.

2. When meeting the patient, the phlebotomist should introduce him- or herself.
   - ○ The introduction should include the phlebotomist's name, title, and reason for the visit.
   - ○ When entering a patient's room, knock gently and open the door slowly.
   - ○ If a provider or clergy is with the patient, wait until they are finished. (If the test is stat or timed, the phlebotomist should politely introduce him- or herself and ask for permission to proceed.)

3. Confirm the patient's identity with two identifiers.
   - ○ Ask the patient to state their full name and date of birth. The patient's response must match the labels and requisition form before the phlebotomist proceeds.
   - ○ Check the **ID bracelet** next and confirm that the information there (**medical record number, patient name, and date of birth**) also matches the requisition form.
   - ○ When the patient cannot confirm their identity (e.g., patient is unconscious, mentally impaired, does not speak English, etc.):
     - · Verify the patient's name and date of birth (DOB) with a nurse, provider, or patient's family member and match this information with wristband ID.
     - · Unconscious patients without ID in the emergency department may have a temporary number/name assigned to them. This will be cross-referenced with a permanent number once their identity can be confirmed.
     - · The ID band is usually found on the leg of patients <2 years old.
   - ○ If a discrepancy is found, notify the patient's nurse. Do not collect specimens until identification is verified and the discrepancy is corrected/addressed.

4. Obtain **patient consent** before specimen collection.
   - ○ **Expressed** consent is given orally or in writing.
   - ○ **Implied consent** is given when the patient's actions imply consent for procedures or when lifesaving care is needed.

- ○ **Informed consent** is given by the patient after they have been educated on the benefits and risks of a procedure.
- ○ Minors (<18 years old) cannot consent to medical procedures. A guardian must provide consent.
- ○ All patients have a **right to refuse consent** for medical procedures.
- ○ Patient refusal should be documented in written form and in the patient's chart.

5. Verify the testing requirements and patient considerations.
   - ○ Verify patient compliance with testing requirements.
   - ○ If the patient has not met the testing requirements, check with the patient's provider to see if the specimen should be collected or rescheduled. Note the issue on the tube if the test is drawn.
   - ○ Does the patient have a **latex allergy**? If so, confirm all equipment is latex-free.
   - ○ Does the patient have a history of **fainting?** If so, place patient in a recliner, supine, or in a chair with a locking arm.
   - ○ Remain calm and professional if the patient appears **anxious**, **agitated**, or **fearful**.

HELPFUL HINT
Fasting means no food or drink for 8 – 12 hours. Most of the time patients can still drink water. *Basal state* refers to the body's metabolic state after fasting for 12 hours or overnight.

QUICK REVIEW QUESTION

5. Before donating blood, a patient sits with the phlebotomist, who explains the procedure and the risks involved. The patient then signs a consent form. What type of consent has the patient given?

Venipuncture Procedures

1. Position the patient for specimen collection.
   - ○ Outpatients should be seated in a phlebotomy chair with an armrest or a recliner.
   - ○ For draws on inpatients, have the patient lie in bed with their arm extended. Do not forget to put bed rails back up after collection.
   - ○ Never have the patient stand or sit on a chair without arms during phlebotomy because of the risk of fainting and falling.
   - ○ For venipuncture in the antecubital area, the patient will need to extend the arm downward and keep the elbow straight.
2. Apply a tourniquet and have the patient make a fist.
   - ○ Apply tourniquet to arm 2 – 4 inches (5 – 10 cm) above the site of intended blood draw to make veins more prominent and easier to select.
   - ○ The tourniquet should be tight enough to restrict venous flow but not occlude arterial flow.
   - ○ Band should lie flat on the skin, not be rolled or twisted.

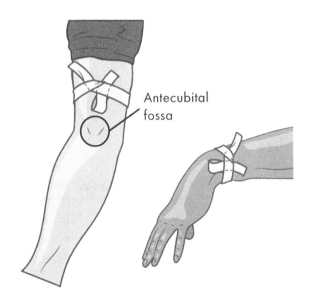

Antecubital fossa

Figure 2.7. Tourniquet for Venipuncture (Antecubital Fossa and Hand)

- The tourniquet ends should point away from the venipuncture site to prevent contamination.
3. Select a site.
   - Venipuncture should be done in the **antecubital (AC) fossa** (the depression in the inside of the elbow).
   - Sites in the forearm, wrist, or hand should only be used if no veins can be accessed in the AC area.
   - Do not use sites that are bruised, infected, burned, edematous, or cyanotic, or sites that have scars or rashes.
   - For patients with **H-pattern** AC veins, the **median cubital vein** is the preferred site. The **cephalic vein** can also be used.
   - For patients with **M-pattern** AC veins, the **median vein** is the preferred site. The **median cephalic vein** can also be used.
   - The **basilic vein** is the last choice for venipuncture in the AC area because it overlies nerves and an artery.

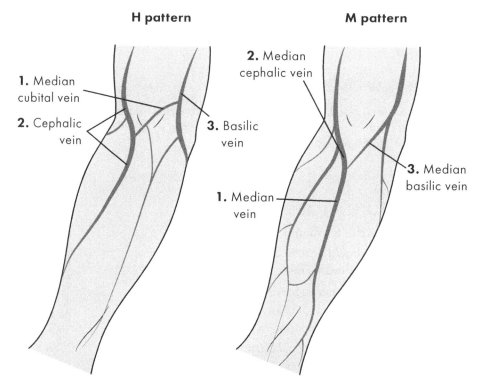

Figure 2.8. Venipuncture Sites in the Antecubital Fossa

   - Palpate the vein by rolling it under an index finger to determine its patency, size, depth, and direction.
   - If the vessel pulses, it is an artery and should be avoided.
   - Once a site has been selected, release the tourniquet and have the patient open their hand.
4. Clean and dry site.
   - Cleanse the site with antiseptic (usually a 70% isopropyl alcohol swab).
   - Start at the site and clean in concentric circles away from the center extending 2 – 3 inches (5 – 7.6 cm) in diameter.

○ Let the site air dry for 30 seconds.

○ Do not fan, touch, or blow on the site while it is drying.

5. Prepare equipment.

○ Review orders and select the appropriate equipment, including needles and collection tubes.

○ Attach needle to collection device.

○ Arrange collection equipment, gauze, and alcohol wipes within reach on phlebotomy tray.

6. Reapply tourniquet.

7. Have patient make a fist and anchor the vein by placing thumb a few centimeters below the site.

8. Insert needle.

○ Align needle along vein with bevel facing upward.

○ For AC venipunctures, enter skin at a 30-degree angle.

○ More superficial veins (like those in the hand) may require a shallower angle of insertion, around 10 degrees.

○ Stop insertion when there is a decrease in resistance (often referred to as a "pop").

9. Establish blood flow, then release tourniquet and ask patient to release fist.

○ If using ETS, advance the collection tube onto the tube holder needle to activate the vacuum. Blood will then fill the tube.

○ If using a syringe system, a flash of blood will be seen in the syringe hub. Then pull slowly back on the plunger to fill the syringe.

10. Fill, remove, and mix tubes.

○ Follow order of draw to prevent additive cross contamination.

○ Tubes should be filled until vacuum is exhausted to ensure the correct additive-to-blood ratio.

○ Invert tubes according to type and manufacturer (typically 3 – 10 inversions).

11. Place gauze, remove needle, and apply pressure.

○ To finish the blood draw, place a folded 2 × 2 in (5 × 5 cm) piece of gauze over the site and draw the needle out of the skin.

12. Activate the needle safety feature and dispose of equipment properly.

13. Label and initial the collected tubes before the patient leaves the room. (See chapter 4 for more information on proper labeling.)

QUICK REVIEW QUESTIONS

6. During which part of the venipuncture procedure should the tourniquet be released from the patient's arm?

7. A patient enters a clinic for a routine CBC. While the patient is in the waiting room, the phlebotomist gathers equipment, including a 20-gauge multi-sample needle, two EDTA tubes, and a tube holder, labels the tubes, and calls the patient back for collection. What mistake(s) did this phlebotomist make while preparing for the blood draw?

HELPFUL HINT
Always remove the tourniquet before removing the needle.

Pediatric Venipuncture

- Pediatric patients may require additional considerations during venipuncture.
- Veins in pediatric patients will be smaller and harder to locate and puncture. Only specially trained phlebotomists should attempt venipuncture on children <2.
- Only small amounts of blood can be drawn safely from pediatric patients.
  - The maximum draw in milliliters for a pediatric patient is roughly twice their weight in kilograms (e.g., the maximum draw from a 6 kg [13.2 lbs] patient is 12 mL).

- Pediatric patients, particularly infants and toddlers, are likely to move during venipuncture and may require **restraints**.
  - Newborns should be swaddled in a blanket.
  - Toddlers and young children should be positioned in a parent's lap (in a bear hug or back-to-chest position).
  - Older children can often sit alone but a parent or provider should be present to steady the arm if needed.
- Parents can play a key role in the anxiety level of the pediatric patient. Keep parents calm and involved in the process.
- A topical anesthetic may be used to reduce pain from venipuncture in children older than 12 months.

QUICK REVIEW QUESTION

8. A phlebotomist needs to do a venipuncture draw on a 3-year-old patient. The patient is excited and restless, refusing to sit in a parent's lap and trying to grab equipment from the phlebotomy cart. What are some techniques the phlebotomist can use to calm the patient for venipuncture?

Geriatric Venipuncture

- Special consideration should be given to **geriatric** patients because of the physical changes to the body caused by aging.
- The skin will be thinner, and may be sagged and wrinkled.
- Vascular changes include:
  - decreased blood flow resulting from impaired peripheral circulation
  - narrowing of blood vessels
  - loss of elasticity in vasculature, making veins more likely to collapse
- Patients who are **blind** or who have **low vision** can be assisted by:
  - having adequate lighting
  - offering to guide the patient to the chair or restroom for specimen collection
  - providing written instructions in a larger print
- Patients who are **deaf** or **hard of hearing** can be assisted by:

- moving closer and facing the patient when speaking to them
- speaking clearly (without shouting) and allowing time for them to answer

- Patients with **mental impairments** (including **dementia**) can be assisted by:
  - being patient and talking slowly
  - allowing extra time for the patient to respond to your question
  - approaching patients calmly and not taking offense if the patient appears hostile or agitated
  - using simple, short statements
- Older patients are more likely to be on medications that affect clotting, putting them at higher risk for excessive bleeding or hematomas.

QUICK REVIEW QUESTION

9. What vascular changes are seen in geriatric patients?

Special Collections and Testing Requirements

- **Blood bank specimens** are used to test for compatibility of donor and recipient blood for transfusions.
  - Blood bank specimens are collected in lavender- or pink-top EDTA tubes.
  - Blood bank specimens have strict labeling requirements to prevent patients from receiving incompatible blood products.
  - Specimens may require specialized blood bank ID barcodes.

Table 2.4. Blood Bank Specimen Tests

Test Name	Tests For . . .
Antibody (Ab) screen	the presence of specific antibodies that are directed against red blood cell antigens
Direct antiglobulin test (DAT)	the presence of antibodies attached to RBCs; used to identify some types of anemia and blood transfusion reactions
Type and crossmatch	patient's blood group (ABO), antibodies in recipient's blood, and compatibility of recipient and donor blood
Type and Rh	patient's blood group (ABO) and type (Rh positive or negative)
Compatibility testing	unsuspected antibodies and antigens in donor or recipient blood by mixing recipient blood with either a donor sample or a sample with a known profile

- During **blood donor collection**, blood is collected from donors for transfusions.
  - Donors must meet the following requirements: be at least 17 years old, be in good health, weigh at least 110 lbs (50 kg), and have a hemoglobin count of 12.5 g/dL and hematocrit of 38%.

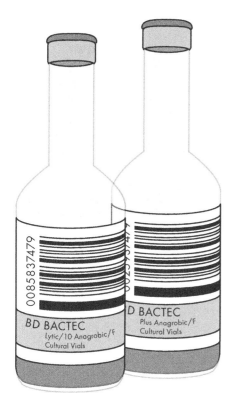

Figure 2.10. Anaerobic and Aerobic Blood Culture Bottles

HELPFUL HINT

Important Considerations for Blood Cultures:

Iodine or chlorohexidine should be used to vigorously clean puncture site.

Collection bottles can only be held at room temperature for up to 4 hours.

Blood cultures should not be collected from central lines or arterial catheters unless venipuncture cannot be done.

Blood cultures are always collected first.

○ The additive **citrate phosphate dextrose (CPD)** is used to preserve blood for transfusions. It includes an anticoagulant and dextrose to preserve RBCs.

○ **Autologous donation** is when a patient donates their own blood preoperatively for a surgery that carries a risk of blood loss.

○ **Cell salvaging** is the recovery of blood lost during surgery, which is reinfused into the patient.

○ Blood is typically collected from the large antecubital vein using procedures similar to routine venipuncture.

○ If the bag does not fill completely, a new unit must be collected; venipuncture cannot be repeated to fill the partially filled unit.

● **Therapeutic phlebotomy** is the removal of large volumes of blood as a medical treatment.

○ The most common disorders that require therapeutic phlebotomy are **polycythemia** (excessive number of RBCs) and **hemochromatosis** (excessive storage of iron).

○ Collection is similar to the procedure for blood donor collection.

● **Blood cultures** and **culture and sensitivity (C&S)** specimens are used to detect the presence and type of bacteria causing an infection so an appropriate antibiotic can be used for treatment.

○ Blood culture specimens are collected in specialized bottles that include additives to promote the growth of bacteria.

○ Multiple blood cultures taken from at least two puncture sites are needed to provide the best chance of identifying pathogens.

○ Each collection should include two bottles: one **aerobic** (with air) and one **anaerobic** (without air).

○ Recommended collection volumes are determined by a patient's weight.

○ **Skin asepsis** (the process of removing all microorganisms from the skin) is essential to prevent normal skin bacteria from contaminating the specimen.

○ Skin should be vigorously rubbed with iodine (or chlorohexidine gluconate for patients with an iodine sensitivity) for 30 – 60 seconds.

● The **oral glucose tolerance test (OGTT)** measures the patient's insulin response to glucose.

○ The patient consumes a drink with a known amount of glucose, and blood glucose draws are then done at regular intervals.

○ The patient must have fasted for at least 8 hours but no more than 16 hours before the test starts.

○ A blood glucose draw may be done before the patient consumes the drink.

○ The timing for the blood glucose draw starts when the patient has finished the drink. For example, if a patient finished the drink at 8:50 a.m. and needs glucose levels checked every half hour, the first draw would be at 9:20 a.m.

○ The number and timing of draws depends on the specific test. Review the requisition order for details.

- An **oral glucose challenge test (OGCT)** is a specialized type of OGTT that tests for gestational diabetes.

- A **2-hour postprandial (2-hour PP)** glucose test is performed on a patient 2 hours after they have eaten a meal.
  - Patients must fast overnight for 10 – 12 hours.
  - Patients may drink a glucose beverage or eat a meal at home.
  - The blood glucose draw is done 2 hours after the drink or meal is finished.

- A **lactose tolerance test** follows the same procedures as a 2-hour GTT, but the patient ingests lactose instead of a glucose drink.

- An **ethanol (ETOH)** test measures the amount of alcohol in the blood. This number can also be used to find the **blood alcohol concentration (BAC)**.
  - ETOH specimens can be collected for medical or legal reasons and should follow chain of custody protocols.
  - Skin should be cleaned with a nonalcoholic antiseptic such as benzalkonium chloride (BZK).
  - Fill a glass gray-top sodium fluoride tube until vacuum is exhausted.

- A **lipid panel** tests levels of fats in the blood, which include cholesterol, triglycerides, low-density lipoproteins (LDL), and high-density lipoproteins (HDL).
  - Patients must fast for 12 hours before a blood draw for a lipid panel.
  - Draws for lipid panels should be done after the patient has been lying or sitting quietly for at least 5 minutes.

- Other tests that require fasting include:
  - vitamin B-12 (fasting time of 6 – 8 hours)
  - iron (fasting time of 12 hours)
  - gamma-glutamyl transferase (GGT) (fasting time of 8 hours)

QUICK REVIEW QUESTIONS

10. A patient presents to the lab for a glucose tolerance test at 7:10 a.m. The patient is given the glucose drink at 7:30 and finishes the drink at 7:45. At what times should the specimens be collected for the 30-minute, 1-hour, 2-hour, and 3-hour tests?

11. A patient comes into a clinic at 8:00 a.m. for a lactose tolerance test. In the waiting room, the phlebotomist notices that the patient is drinking orange juice. What should the phlebotomist do?

12. When blood is collected for the purpose of blood transfusion, the additive CPD (citrate phosphate dextrose) is present in the collection bag. What is the purpose of this additive?

Patient Considerations for Venipuncture

- A **mastectomy** is a surgical breast removal.
  - Mastectomy may include the removal of lymph nodes that drain lymph from the affected arm.

○ Drawing blood from the same side as a mastectomy puts the patient at risk for **lymphedema**, extreme swelling caused by a buildup of lymph that may damage the sample.

○ Do not draw blood from the arm on the same side as the mastectomy without consulting the patient's physician.

Normal

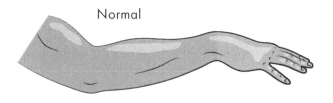

Lymphedema

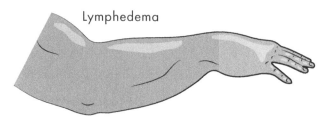

Figure 2.11. Lymphedema in the Arm

• **Venous access devices (VADs)** provide constant access to a patient's vein or artery.

○ VADs include IV lines, IV catheter locks, arterial lines, and central vascular access devices (CVADs).

○ Blood can be drawn directly from VADs; however, most of these specimens must be collected by a nurse.

○ When specimens are collected from devices flushed with heparin, a 5 mL discard tube should be drawn first.

○ Blood should never be collected from a fistula or graft.

• **Intravenous (IV) lines** are used to administer fluids, medications, and blood transfusions.

○ IV lines may be placed in the arm, wrist, or hand.

○ Fluid and medications from IV lines may contaminate blood specimens.

○ Do not perform venipuncture on the same side as the patient's IV unless no other site is available.

○ If a draw must be performed on an arm with an IV:

· Draw distal to (below) the IV site.

· Have the nurse turn off IV medications for at least 2 minutes prior to collection. Make sure that nurse restarts medication when draw is complete.

· Apply tourniquet below the IV site.

○ Do not collect from a previous IV site for 24 – 48 hours after the IV has been removed.

- Veins in an **obese patient** can be more difficult to visualize or find.
  - Use a **bariatric tourniquet** if possible; these are longer than standard tourniquets.
  - An extra-large blood pressure cuff can be inflated to just below the patient's diastolic blood pressure level if the appropriate tourniquet is not available.
  - Try to palpate the median cubital vein in the AC area or the cephalic vein with the wrist prone.
- **Dehydration** is an excessive loss of fluids from the body.
  - Dehydration can be caused by lifestyle factors (e.g., exercising in the heat) or medical conditions (e.g., excessive vomiting or urination).
  - Dehydration may lead to **hemoconcentration**, abnormally high concentrations of some blood components.
  - Labs affected by dehydration include RBCs, enzymes, iron, calcium, sodium, and clotting factors.
  - Fasting patients should be encouraged to drink water (when allowed) to avoid dehydration.
- **Damaged veins** feel cord-like and hard.
  - Causes of damaged veins include blood clots, atherosclerosis, and scarring caused by frequent venipuncture.
  - Avoid drawing blood from damaged veins if possible.
  - Draw distal to damaged veins if no other sites are suitable.
- **Edema** is swelling that occurs when fluid leaks out of blood vessels and into surrounding tissue.
  - Do not collect blood from edematous areas; the specimen may be contaminated by tissue fluid.
  - Veins are often more difficult to locate in edematous tissue and may be more fragile.
- Avoid drawing from **paralyzed** extremities when possible.
  - Lack of muscle movement can decrease blood flow and lead to thrombosis; this risk is increased by venipuncture.
  - The patient may also be unable to feel adverse reactions to venipuncture.

QUICK REVIEW QUESTIONS

13. A phlebotomist needs to draw a sample for a liver panel from a patient with IV lines in both arms. How should the sample be collected?

14. A patient who has had a double mastectomy comes to a clinic for an oral glucose challenge test. How should the phlebotomist choose a site for venipuncture?

Venipuncture Complications

- **Syncope** describes fainting or loss of consciousness from insufficient blood flow to the brain.

- Syncope can happen before, during, or after venipuncture as part of a nervous system response to stress.
- Always ask patient about prior syncopal or near-fainting episodes. If they have occurred, have the patient supine or reclined for the procedure.
- Signs that a patient might faint include pallor, sweating, rapid breathing, and unsteadiness or loss of motor control.
- If a patient is showing signs they might faint:
    - Release tourniquet, stop venipuncture, and discard sharp.
    - Apply pressure to site of blood draw.
    - Have patient lower their head and take deep breaths.
    - Distract the patient by talking with them.
    - Support the patient to prevent them from falling.
    - Apply cool compress to back of the neck or forehead.
    - Do not leave the patient alone until they recover.

- **Nausea** or **vomiting** may happen during blood draw or before syncopal episode.
    - Stop blood draw immediately.
    - Provide patient with emesis bag, basin, or trashcan.
    - Apply cool compress to back of the neck or forehead.

- **Needle phobia** is an extreme fear of needles.
    - Be empathetic and calm.
    - Position the patient supine to prevent fainting if possible.
    - Place an ice pack on venipuncture site for 10 – 15 minutes before lab draw to decrease sensation and pain from needlestick.

- A **seizure** is caused by abnormal electrical discharges in the brain that disrupt normal brain function. Seizures may include rapid, uncontrolled contraction of muscles.
    - If a seizure occurs, stop blood draw immediately.
    - Hold pressure on site without restraining the patient.
    - Lower patient to the floor and turn them onto their side for airway protection.
    - Place padding under their head and remove dangerous objects from the area around the patient.

- Rapid breathing and situational anxiety can lead to **hyperventilation**.
    - Patients will often report tingling around the mouth or fingertips.
    - Attempt to calm the patient and address their concerns or anxiety.
    - Stop blood draw until the patient is calm and ready to proceed.

- **Iatrogenic anemia** results from too much blood being collected too frequently.
    - Greater than 10% blood volume loss can be life threatening.
    - **NICU infants** are at particularly high risk.
    - Iatrogenic anemia can be prevented by collecting the least amount of blood necessary and minimizing redraws.
    - NICU blood transfusions are sometimes given to compensate for blood loss from frequent blood draws.

- More than 5 minutes of bleeding despite pressure application on puncture site is considered **excessive bleeding**.
  - Medications (e.g., warfarin, prednisone, naproxen, aspirin) can prolong bleeding times.
  - If bleeding lasts more than 5 minutes, notify a supervisor or the patient's provider.
  - Do not apply a pressure bandage and dismiss a patient until bleeding has stopped.
- A **hematoma** is painful swelling and bruising at the phlebotomy site from blood rapidly leaking into the tissue.
  - Causes of hematoma include:
    - injury to artery or vein
    - needle too large or inserted incorrectly
    - removal of needle while tourniquet still in place
    - inadequate pressure on blood draw site after needle was removed
    - folding the elbow immediately after venipuncture
  - Patients can be advised to take over-the-counter pain medication and apply ice to puncture site if a painful hematoma develops.
  - If hematoma develops during blood draw:
    - Stop blood draw immediately to prevent further injury.
    - Hold pressure on the site for 3 – 5 minutes or until bleeding stops.
    - If the hematoma is large, elevate the patient's arm over their head.
    - Do not attempt additional lab draws at this site.
- **Petechiae** are small amounts of blood that leak from the capillaries into the skin surface.
  - They appear as tiny, flat, red or purple skin spots, <3 mm in diameter.
  - Petechiae can be caused by:
    - overly tight tourniquet
    - capillary wall defect
    - platelet abnormality or delayed clotting time
    - medications that prolong clotting time (e.g., aspirin, warfarin)
    - infection or inflammatory disease
  - Petechiae can suggest the patient will bleed excessively.
  - If petechiae appear during draw, check that the tourniquet is not overly tight.
- **Nerve injury** can result in permanent loss of motor or sensory function of the extremity.
  - Nerves may be directly damaged by a needle or compressed by pooling blood or a tourniquet.
  - Signs of nerve injury include:
    - extreme pain, often radiating up and down the arm
    - a burning or electric shock sensation
    - tingling or numbness
  - If a nerve injury is suspected:

- Stop venipuncture immediately and remove the needle.
- Apply ice pack to reduce inflammation.
- Document the incident and report it to the patient's provider.

- An accidental **arterial puncture** can lead to compression injury if a large hematoma develops.
  - Arterial punctures are usually caused by blind or deep probing.
  - Arterial punctures occur most often in the brachial artery because it is near the basilic vein.
  - Signs of an arterial puncture include:
    - rapid development of a hematoma
    - blood filling tube quickly
    - blood that is pulsatile or bright red
  - If an arterial puncture is suspected:
    - Stop blood draw immediately.
    - Apply direct forceful pressure until bleeding stops (usually 3 – 5 minutes).
    - Identify specimen as possible arterial blood.

- **Reflux of blood** occurs when blood in the tube or tubing flows back into the patient's vein.
  - Reflux can be caused by a normal variation in vein pressure or by a drop in pressure from tourniquet release.
  - If the contents of the tube contact the needle, any additive in the tube may reflux into the vein. This can cause an adverse or allergic reaction.
  - To prevent **additive reflux**, keep the patient's arm down and hold the tube still below venipuncture site.

QUICK REVIEW QUESTIONS

15. What life-threatening complication can result from frequent phlebotomy to infants?

16. A patient preparing for venipuncture states that she's nervous because she passed out the last time she had blood drawn. What precautions should the phlebotomist take with this patient?

Failure to Draw Blood

- Failure to obtain blood during a venipuncture can be caused by failure of technique or equipment.

- Incorrect needle position can lead to failure of blood flow.

- Problems with the tube may also prevent adequate blood flow.
  - The tube may be improperly positioned.
  - The tube's vacuum may be defective.
  - Correct by repositioning. If that does not work, try a new tube.

Table 2.5. Troubleshooting Needle Position During Venipuncture

Cause	Signs	Response
needle too shallow (not in vein)	no blood flow	Insert needle deeper.
needle too deep (through vein)	one spurt of blood, then no blood flow	Pull needle out until blood flow is established.
bevel out of skin	no blood flow; hiss as vacuum escapes tube	Insert needle deeper; discard used tube.
bevel partially out of vein	slow blood flow; formation of hematoma	Reposition needle so that bevel is within the vein; remove needle if a hematoma has formed.
bevel against vein wall	no blood flow	This is commonly caused by shallow angle of insertion; release the tube from holder and reposition the needle.
needle outside vein	lack of "pop"; no blood flow	Release tube, withdraw the needle slightly, and redirect the needle into the vein.

- A collapsed vein will prevent adequate blood flow.

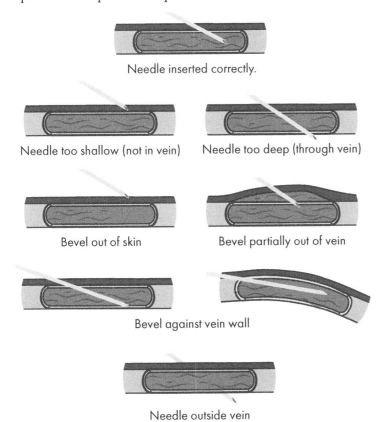

Needle inserted correctly.

Needle too shallow (not in vein)　　Needle too deep (through vein)

Bevel out of skin　　Bevel partially out of vein

Bevel against vein wall

Needle outside vein

Figure 2.12. Needle Position and Potential Causes of Failure to Draw Blood

- If a vein collapses, it will become invisible when the tube vacuum engages.
- Causes of collapsed veins include a tourniquet that is too tight, a vacuum that is too strong, or a tourniquet placed too close to the venipuncture site.
- To correct a collapsed vein:
  - Attempt to adjust/reapply tourniquet to increase pressure.
  - Apply pressure to the vein with finger several inches proximal to (above) needle site.
  - Remove tube and wait for blood flow to return for second attempt.
  - Use a smaller-volume tube.

QUICK REVIEW QUESTION

17. While drawing labs on a patient, the phlebotomist notices a flash of blood, but then the tube does not appear to be filling. What could be the cause and what should the phlebotomist do next?

Skin Puncture Equipment

- During **skin (capillary) puncture**, a small amount of blood is collected from capillaries by cutting or puncturing the skin.

- Skin punctures may be used in the following situations:
  - newborn screening (NBS)
  - point-of-care testing (e.g., blood glucose monitoring)
  - adults who are not eligible for venipuncture (if test can be done on capillary specimen)

- Some tests usually done with a venipuncture sample may be done with a capillary sample if necessary. These include:
  - CBC
  - hemoglobin and hematocrit (H&H)
  - electrolytes
  - glucose and hemoglobin A1c
  - lipids

Table 2.6. Common Skin Puncture Tests

Test Name	Tests For . . .	Special Considerations
Capillary blood gas (CBG)	pH and levels of O_2 and CO_2 in the blood (CBG is an alternative to arterial blood gases because arterial punctures are too hazardous for infants.)	Minimize exposure of capillary blood gas specimens to air; oxygen in the air can alter the gas composition of the sample.
Bilirubin (neonatal)	bilirubin levels, which will be elevated if the liver is not functioning properly or if red blood cell hemolysis is occurring	Bilirubin specimens are sensitive to light and should be collected in amber containers. Neonatal bilirubin is a timed test measured from time of birth.

Test Name	Tests For ...	Special Considerations
Newborn screening	genetic, metabolic, hormonal, and functional disorders in newborns that can cause disabilities if not detected and treated early four mandatory tests: phenylketonuria (PKU), cystic fibrosis (CF), hypothyroidism, and galactosemia (GALT)	Blood drops are placed on circles on special filter paper. Required screening tests vary by state.
Blood smear	manual **differential** (a count of the number, type, and characteristics of blood cells done through a microscope)	Blood drop is thinly spread onto microscope slide.
Thick blood smear	malaria (caused by a blood parasite), which can cause severe anemia	Spread the blood into a circle about the size of a dime, dry the slide for 2 hours, and apply **Giemsa stain**.

- A **lancet** is an instrument with a retractable blade used to puncture the skin on the fingertip (or heel for an infant) to obtain a capillary blood specimen.

- **Microcollection containers** (or **microtubes**) are small plastic tubes designed to collect small amounts of blood following capillary puncture.
  - Tubes are color-coded as for ETS.
  - Typical capacity is 250 – 500 microliters (μL).
  - If venous blood is obtained via syringe and placed into a microtube, it should be labeled "venous."

- **Microhematocrit tubes** are used to collect specimens for hematocrit levels.
  - Typical capacity is 50 – 75 μL.
  - Colored bands indicate additive type (green and red: heparin; blue: nonadditive).

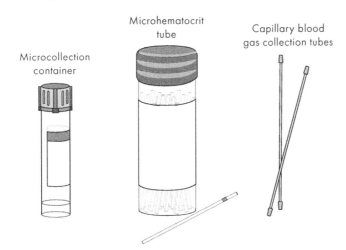

Microhematocrit tube

Capillary blood gas collection tubes

Microcollection container

Figure 2.13. Capillary Puncture Collection Devices

- **Capillary blood gas (CBG) collection tubes** are long, thin plastic tubes lined with heparin.
  - ○ A magnet and stirrer can be used to mix the anticoagulant.
  - ○ The most commonly used CBG tubes are 100 mm (4 in) in length and have a 100 μL capacity.

QUICK REVIEW QUESTION

18. A phlebotomist needs to collect a CBC specimen from a patient with an IV line in the right arm and significant bruising on the AC region of the left arm. How should the phlebotomist collect the sample?

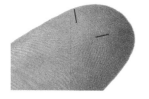

Figure 2.14. Location of Finger-Stick

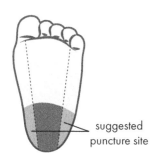

suggested puncture site

Figure 2.15. Infant Heel Puncture Site

HELPFUL HINT

Important Considerations for Skin Punctures:

Puncture skin perpendicular to fingerprint lines.

Maximum depth of puncture for infant heel sticks is 2 mm.

Wipe away the first drop of blood before collecting the sample.

Never touch newborn screening filter paper to the neonate's skin.

Never do a skin puncture at the site of a previous puncture.

Do not use povidone-iodine for skin puncture.

Skin Puncture Procedures

1. Position the patient.
   - ○ finger puncture: arm extended with palm facing upward
   - ○ heel puncture: hold infant supine with foot lower than the body
2. Select the site.
   - ○ For a finger puncture, the medial or lateral side of the middle or ring finger is preferred.
     - · Do not perform puncture on nail, thumb, little finger, or middle of the finger pad.
     - · Puncture site should be perpendicular to the fingerprint lines of the middle or ring fingertip.
   - ○ For a heel puncture on an infant, choose the medial or lateral side of heel, or the big toe if necessary.
3. Warm the site to increase blood flow and quicken collection time.
   - ○ Wrap the site for 3 – 5 minutes with a warm towel, washcloth, or heel warming device.
   - ○ Do not squeeze or compress the site—this may compromise the sample.
4. Clean site with an antiseptic and allow to dry.
   - ○ Use an antiseptic such as a 70% isopropyl alcohol swab.
   - ○ Start at the site and clean in concentric circles away from center, extending 2 – 3 inches in diameter.
   - ○ Let site air dry for 30 seconds.
   - ○ Do not fan, touch, or blow on the site while it is drying.
   - ○ Do not use povidone-iodine for skin puncture. It can interfere with bilirubin, uric acid, phosphorous, and potassium level testing.
5. Choose equipment (including collection tubes, gauze, and lancet) and place within reach.
   - ○ For infant heel puncture, prepare equipment with guardian present.
   - ○ Wash hands and put on gloves, if not already done.
6. Grasp site of puncture (finger or heel) with nondominant hand.
   - ○ For a finger puncture, hold three or four of patient's fingers between fingers and thumb. (Holding only one finger allows it to slip out more easily.)

○ For a heel puncture, grasp the patient's foot by stabilizing the heel with thumb and index fingers; the remaining fingers wrap around the top of the foot.

7. Puncture the skin.
   ○ Position the lancet perpendicular to and flush against the skin without applying too much pressure or pressing too deeply.
   ○ Warn patient or parent prior to puncture.
   ○ Press lancet release mechanism to puncture skin.
   ○ The maximum skin puncture depth is 2 mm.

8. Discard lancet in sharps container.

9. Apply pressure until blood appears.
   ○ Wipe away the first drop of blood to prevent contamination from tissue fluid or residue from antiseptic.
   ○ Hold extremity facing downward and gently apply pressure toward puncture site to promote bleeding.
   ○ Do not squeeze puncture site with too much force; this will cause hemolysis.

10. Keep finger or heel downward and intermittently gently massage to fill collection device.
    ○ Fill tubes and containers in order of draw by touching collection tubes or slides to drop of blood.
    ○ Order of draw for capillary specimens (per CLSI):
      1. blood gas
      2. EDTA/anticoagulant
      3. other additives
      4. serum
    ○ Complete newborn screening test by touching the filter paper to the blood from the heel puncture until the entire circle is filled.

11. Place gauze, apply pressure, and elevate site until bleeding stops.

12. Label specimens.

13. Apply bandage after rechecking site.
    ○ Notify supervisor or provider if bleeding persists for more than 5 minutes.
    ○ Bandages can often be removed after 15 minutes.

QUICK REVIEW QUESTIONS

19. During a heel puncture, the phlebotomist aggressively massaged an infant's foot to express blood after puncturing the center of the heel. What levels could be affected?

20. A phlebotomist needs to draw one lavender-top and one red-top microcollection container from a capillary puncture. Which container should be drawn first?

Answer Key

1. The size and type of needle is dependent on patient age, quality of veins, and type of collection needed.
   a) A **15- to 17-gauge needle** is used for blood donation.
   b) A **23-gauge butterfly** is typically used for hand veins in adults.
   c) A **25-gauge butterfly** is usually used for premature and neonate scalp veins.
   d) A **21-gauge multi-sample** is the standard venipuncture needle for patients with normal-sized veins.

2. The order of draw recommended by CLSI is:
   1. blood cultures
   2. sodium citrate tubes
   3. serum tubes
   4. heparin tubes
   5. EDTA tubes
   6. sodium fluoride/potassium oxalate

   The phlebotomist should draw **1) the citrate tube, then 2) the SST, and then 3) the PPT (an EDTA tube)**.

3. A diagnosis of anemia is confirmed by a CBC, which measures levels of RBCs and hemoglobin (the iron-containing protein that transports oxygen in the blood). CBC specimens are collected in EDTA (lavender) tubes.

4. An antiseptic (e.g., isopropyl alcohol) prevents the growth of microorganisms but does not kill them. A disinfectant (e.g., bleach) will kill microorganisms. Phlebotomists use antiseptics to clean a patient's skin before a puncture, and they use disinfectants to clean surfaces that may have come in contact with bodily fluids.

5. The patient has given informed, written consent. The patient was advised of the procedures and risks involved in blood donation and signed a written consent form.

6. The tourniquet is applied and released twice during venipuncture. The tourniquet should be applied to help with site selection. Once the site has been selected, the tourniquet is released. The tourniquet is then reapplied before the needle is inserted. It should be removed once blood flow is established and before the needle is removed.

7. Equipment should be collected after the phlebotomist has examined the veins and selected a site for venipuncture. In addition, tubes should be labeled after the collection has been drawn.

8. The phlebotomist should be warm and calm toward the patient and the parents. They might ask the parents for input about past venipunctures and techniques that have worked for their child. A 3-year-old can understand basic instructions, so the phlebotomist can explain in very simple terms what is about to happen. The patient can be placed in a parent's lap in a bear hug or back-to-chest position for the draw.

9. Blood vessels in geriatric patients may have slower or decreased blood flow from impaired peripheral circulation. They may also be narrowed or hardened due to atherosclerosis, scarring, or thrombosis. The loss of elasticity may make veins more prone to collapsing.

10. The clock starts when the patient has finished drinking the glucose drink (7:45 a.m. in this case). Thus, tests will be collected at 8:15, 8:45, 9:45, and 10:45 a.m.

11. Patients who are completing a lactose tolerance test should fast for at least 8 hours before the baseline draw. The phlebotomist should notify the patient's provider to see if the test should still be completed if the patient has not fasted. If the test is done, the phlebotomist should write "non-fasting" on the collection tube labels.

12. It is important that blood collected for transfusion does not clot and the cells remain viable for the patient who is receiving the transfusion. The citrate prevents clotting via chelation. The phosphate stabilizes the pH. The dextrose provides nourishment for RBCs to keep them alive longer.

13. The phlebotomist should attempt to collect a sample at a site distal (below) one of the IV lines. Venipuncture should be attempted before a nurse is asked to collect a sample through an IV. A liver panel specimen cannot be collected through capillary puncture.

14. The phlebotomist should contact the patient's provider so they can choose an acceptable site. The phlebotomist should not draw without consulting with the provider.

15. Iatrogenic anemia results from too much blood being taken too frequently, before the patient's body can create new blood cells. This can be prevented by collecting the least amount of blood necessary and minimizing redraws. Infants, particularly those born prematurely, are at risk of iatrogenic anemia from frequent phlebotomy.

16. The phlebotomist should have the patient lie down for the collection and should closely monitor the patient's status during the draw. The phlebotomist should look for signs that may indicate the patient is about to faint, such as pallor, sweating, or disorientation.

17. The bevel likely went completely through the vein. Slowly withdraw the needle until blood flow reestablishes. The phlebotomist should monitor for a hematoma and stop the draw if one appears.

18. A CBC specimen can be quickly and easily taken from a capillary puncture when no vein is easily accessible. The phlebotomist should follow capillary puncture procedures and use an EDTA microtube for collection.19.   Squeezing the tissues too aggressively can cause RBC hemolysis, which can elevate levels of potassium, ammonia, iron, magnesium, and phosphate.

20. The order of draw for a capillary puncture is:
    1. blood gas
    2. EDTA/anticoagulant
    3. other additives
    4. serum

    The lavender-top tube is an EDTA microtube, so it should be collected first.

THREE: NON-BLOOD SPECIMEN COLLECTION

Urine

- **Urine** can be used to test for a wide variety of conditions, including infections, metabolic disorders (e.g., diabetes), organ dysfunction, and cancers, as well as pregnancy.

Table 3.1. Common Tests Performed on Urine

Test Name	Tests For . . .	Type of Specimen
urinalysis (UA)	a variety of substances and conditions: Urine is **physically** inspected for color, amount, clarity, and odor. A **chemical** test (usually using a dipstick) detects bacteria, protein, or blood in the urine. It also tests values such as specific gravity and pH. A **microscopic** analysis reveals the presence and number of particles viewable under a microscope, such as microorganisms, cells, crystals, and casts. (See chapter 4 for details on point-of-care urinalysis.)	random
urine culture and sensitivity (C&S)	microorganisms that cause infection	clean-catch
urine cytology	cancer in the urinary tract	clean-catch (not first morning)
drug screening	presence of drugs	random
pregnancy test	presence of human chorionic gonadotropin (hCG), which indicates pregnancy	first morning

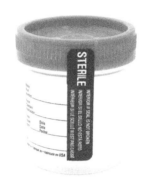

Figure 3.1. Urine Specimen Cup

- Urine samples can be collected in the laboratory, at the provider's office, or in the patient's home.
- Most urine samples are **voided** (passed from the body).
- Collection containers for urinalysis can vary in shape and size but should be labeled and have a tight-fitting lid.
- Some urine collection containers may include a **preservative**. Common preservatives are acetic acid, boric acid, hydrochloric acid, and oxalic acid.
- Urine can be collected at random times or at a specific time.
  - **Random** urine samples are not taken at a scheduled time.
  - Drug screenings are often intentionally randomized. Patients are notified that they have 4 to 6 hours to come to the lab and provide a urine sample.
  - A **first morning** urine sample is collected before the patient takes in any fluid so that the urine is more concentrated.
    - It is usually collected after 8 hours of sleep.
    - If the patient has an unusual sleep cycle, they can be instructed to collect the first urine after any 8-hour period during which they did not urinate.
  - A **timed** urinalysis can span 2 to 72 hours. (A 24-hour specimen is the most common.)
    - Timed tests are usually done when the substance being tested for is excreted at differing rates throughout the day (e.g., testosterone or creatinine).
    - Urine is collected over the given time period and added to a large collection container.
    - The patient should discard their first morning urine and start collecting urine after that.
    - Specimens may be tested for markers such as creatinine or 4-aminobenzoic acid (PABA) to ensure that all urine from the timed period was collected.
  - A **postprandial** test is a timed urine test for glucose done 2 hours after the patient eats.
  - A **fasting** urinalysis tests for glucose after at least 8 hours of fasting.
    - It is usually done first thing in the morning to make it easier on the patient.
    - The patient should discard their first morning urine and collect the second voided urine sample after the fasting period has ended.
- Different collection methods are appropriate for different tests being performed.
  - A **regular voided sample** can be collected by the patient without any special preparations.
  - A **midstream sample** is collected after the patient has voided a small amount of urine to flush material away from the urinary opening.
  - **Double voiding** requires the patient to discard their first morning urine and wait a set amount of time (usually 30 minutes) to collect a sample.

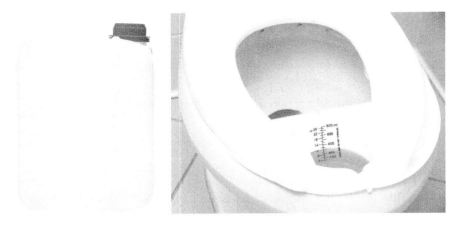
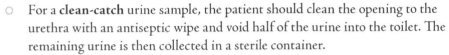

Figure 3.2. Urine Collection Container and Collection Hat for 24-Hour Sample

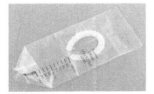

Figure 3.3. Pediatric Collection Bag

- For a **clean-catch** urine sample, the patient should clean the opening to the urethra with an antiseptic wipe and void half of the urine into the toilet. The remaining urine is then collected in a sterile container.
- **Urinary collection bags** are used to collect urine samples from pediatric patients. The adhesive bag is sealed around the baby's genitals and removed once enough urine has been collected.
- **Catheterized** urine samples are collected with a catheter (a tube that is passed through the urethra into the bladder).
- **Suprapubic aspiration** is performed by a physician with local anesthesia when an uncontaminated urine sample is needed. A needle is inserted into the bladder through the abdomen and urine is aspirated into a sterile syringe.

HELPFUL HINT

Taking a urine sample from the tubing of an indwelling catheter is preferable to taking it from the collection bag.

QUICK REVIEW QUESTIONS

1. How long does a patient need to fast before they can provide a fasting urine sample?

2. A phlebotomist is instructing a patient who will be collecting a 24-hour urine sample. When asked to repeat the instructions, the patient says, "I will pee first thing in the morning into the collection hat and set a timer for 24 hours. That urine goes into the collection container, which I'll store in the refrigerator. Then I collect all my urine and immediately pour it into the container until the timer goes off." Which step should the phlebotomist correct?

Stool

- **Stool (fecal) samples** are collected to test for disorders of the gastrointestinal (GI) system, including infections, cancers, and bleeding.
- **Fecal occult blood tests** (also called guaiac tests or guaiac smears) are a common test for occult (hidden) blood. Occult blood may be present if the patient has a GI disorder such as colorectal cancer or ulcerative colitis.
- Stool samples may be collected in a large container placed inside the toilet.

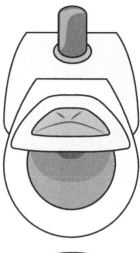

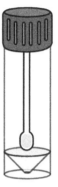

Figure 3.4. Stool Sample Collection Devices

- For smaller samples, the patient may use a scoop to place a small portion of feces in the collection container.

- Special instructions for a patient providing a stool sample for a fecal occult blood test:
  - ○ The patient should not take any NSAIDs, aspirin, or steroids for 1 week before giving a sample.
  - ○ The patient should not take vitamin C or iron for 3 days before collecting a sample.
  - ○ The patient should avoid a number of foods, including red meat, broccoli, cauliflower, turnips, radishes, and melons, for 3 days before collecting a sample. (Consuming these could result in a false positive test.)
  - ○ The patient should not provide a fecal sample if they have a bladder infection, are menstruating, or have bleeding hemorrhoids. (These conditions could result in a false positive test.)

- Fecal tests evaluate stool in three ways:
  - ○ **physical** evaluation for odor, consistency, color, shape, and the presence of any substances like mucus or blood.
  - ○ **chemical** tests, such as tests for the presence of blood or mucus
  - ○ **microscopic** tests, such as the ova and parasite (O&P) test, for the presence of parasites and their eggs, also called ova

Table 3.2. Common Tests Performed on Stool Samples

Test Name	Tests For . . .
guaiac smear	blood originating in the lower GI tract
ova and parasite (O&P)	parasites and their eggs
Cologuard®	altered DNA and biomarkers present with colorectal cancer
immunochemical fecal occult blood test	the globulin portion of hemoglobin
fecal fat test	the presence of fat to diagnose malabsorption
culture and sensitivity	the presence of bacteria such as *C. difficile*

QUICK REVIEW QUESTION

3. What substances can cause an inaccurate result in a fecal test?

Breath

- **Breath samples** are collected by having patients blow into a collection container, usually a specialized bag.

- For a **breathalyzer** test, the patient breathes forcefully into a disposable mouthpiece attached to a testing machine.

- For a **C-urea breath test**, the patient blows into a specialized bag before drinking a solution of synthetic urea. After the drink, the patient waits 15 minutes and then blows into a second bag.

Table 3.3. Common Tests Performed on Breath Samples

Test Name	Tests For . . .
breathalyzer	alcohol
C-urea breath test	carbon-13, which is produced by *H. pylori* (a cause of stomach ulcers)
hydrogen breath test	hydrogen (a side effect of lactose intolerance)

- The **hydrogen breath test** also uses specialized collection bags.
    - The patient breathes into the bag to provide a baseline breath sample.
    - The patient then drinks a solution of lactose or fructose.
    - Breath samples are then taken every 30 minutes for a set length of time (up to 3 hours).
    - Patients must follow a specific diet for the hydrogen breath test:
        - 12-hour fast
        - minimal carbohydrates in the 24 hours before the test
        - no antibiotics for 2 – 4 weeks before the test (depending on provider)
        - no laxatives for 7 days before the test
        - no smoking for 1 hour before the test

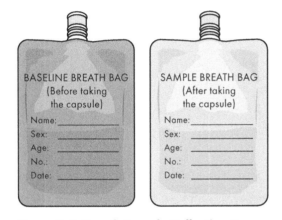

Figure 3.5. Breath Sample Collection Bags

QUICK REVIEW QUESTION

4. What does a positive C-urea breath test indicate?

Swabs

- A **swab** is a piece of absorbent material at the end of a short stick.

- Collections done with swabs include:
    - buccal (or oral)
    - nasopharyngeal (NP)
    - throat

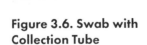

Figure 3.6. Swab with Collection Tube

Table 3.4. Common Tests Performed with Swabs

Test Name	Tests For . . .
DNA analysis (buccal swab)	DNA for forensic and paternity testing; also used to test for genetic predictors of disease
nasopharyngeal culture	influenza, meningitis, pertussis, diphtheria, and pneumonia
throat culture	streptococcal infection

HELPFUL HINT

Chain of custody protocols should be followed for most specimens collected for DNA analysis.

- **Buccal swabs** are done by scraping the cheek or another part of the mouth with a special brush or swab.
- **Nasopharyngeal swabs** are done with a flexible wire or plastic swab.
  - With the patient's head tilted back, the phlebotomist gently inserts the swab into one nostril until it is halfway up the nasal canal and then twists it in a circle to collect a sample.
- **Throat swabs** are done with one or two swabs. Two swabs are usually used when doing a rapid strep test.

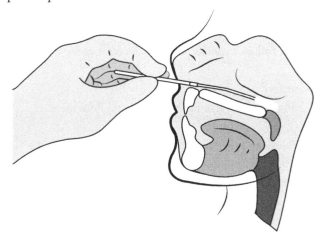

Figure 3.7. Nasopharyngeal Swab Collection

QUICK REVIEW QUESTION

5. A paternity test requires the phlebotomist to collect DNA with what kind of swab?

Oral Fluid (Saliva)

- **Oral fluid (saliva) tests** are done to check hormone levels and reveal the presence of drugs and alcohol.
- Oral fluid tests are usually point-of-care tests, but some can be sent to a lab for confirmation of the results.

- Patients may be asked to spit into special collection containers, or the phlebotomist may use a special collection sponge that is placed in the patient's mouth.

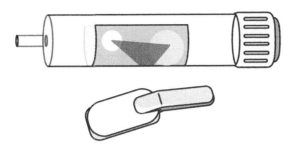

Figure 3.8. Oral Fluid Collection Device

HELPFUL HINT

Special Considerations for Oral Hormone Tests:

The patient should not use certain antiaging creams for at least 3 days before the test.

The patient should also avoid eating, drinking, and brushing their teeth for 2 hours before collecting a sample.

- **Oral hormone** tests measure hormones in the body such as cortisol, estrogen, and testosterone.
  - They are often performed on women with symptoms related to the menstrual cycle or menopause.
  - They typically need to be done 30 minutes after waking in the morning and sometimes intermittently throughout the day.
  - They are frequently done by the patient at home.
  - The patient may be given different colored tubes to be used at different times of day.
  - Samples should be refrigerated or frozen if they will not be processed within 24 hours.

QUICK REVIEW QUESTION

6. A physician is considering hormone replacement therapy for a patient going through menopause and wants to check the patient's current hormone levels. What test will the doctor likely order, and what type of specimen will the phlebotomist collect?

Other Non-Blood Samples

- **Cerebrospinal fluid (CSF)** is a clear liquid that circulates within the central nervous system.
  - CSF specimens may be tested for infections (e.g., meningitis), cancers, and multiple sclerosis.
  - A CSF specimen is obtained during a **lumbar puncture** (spinal tap), in which a physician inserts a needle between the vertebra to extract fluid from the intervertebral space.
  - Specimens are collected in screw-top tubes that are numbered according to the order in which they are collected.
  - The samples must be transported immediately at room temperature to the lab for analysis so that the procedure does not have to be redone.

- If testing cannot be done immediately, serology tubes can be frozen for storage, hematology tubes can be refrigerated, and microbiology tubes can be stored at room temperature for less than 24 hours.
- Samples older than 24 hours will be deemed unacceptable for testing by the laboratory.

- **Amniotic fluid** surrounds a fetus in the uterus.
  - Amniotic fluid is tested for signs of fetal abnormalities (e.g., chromosome disorders and neural tube defects) and gestational age.
  - The fluid is obtained through an **amniocentesis**, during which the physician inserts a needle through the abdomen and into the amniotic sac.
  - An amniocentesis is typically done between weeks 15 and 18 of pregnancy.
  - Amniotic fluid should be stored in a sterile container and protected from exposure to light.
  - It should be brought to the lab for analysis immediately after it is obtained.
  - Samples meant for chromosomal abnormality tests must be kept at room temperature, while samples for chemical analysis must be stored on ice.
  - During labor, amniotic fluid can also be tested for fetal lung maturity.

- **Gastric fluid** is stomach acid that is obtained by aspiration through a nasogastric tube.
  - A baseline reading of the gastric fluid is done after the patient has fasted.
  - After the patient takes a dose of medication to stimulate gastric production, several more samples are aspirated at timed intervals and evaluated for acidity.
  - The phlebotomist typically needs to draw blood samples during the procedures.

- **Serous fluid** is found within the double-layered membranes that surround the pericardial, pleural, and peritoneal cavities.
  - The volume of serous fluid increases during an infection.
  - Serous fluid is collected by a physician using a large needle.
  - The type of serous fluid collection tube used depends on the test ordered.
    - Sterile tubes are used for cultures.
    - Heparin or sodium fluoride tubes are used for chemistry tests.
    - Nonanticoagulant tubes are used for biochemical tests.
    - Tubes containing **EDTA**, a chemical used to prevent cell adhesion, are used for cell counts or smears.
  - Samples should be labeled according to the body cavity they were collected from and the type of test they are intended for.

- **Synovial fluid** cushions and lubricates joints.
  - Its volume increases with infection or injury.
  - It can be removed from joints through needle aspiration to relieve pain or to diagnosis the cause of inflammation (e.g., septic arthritis or gout).
  - The type of tube used depends on the test ordered.
    - A sterile tube is used to collect specimens for diagnosing an infectious process.

- A nonadditive tube is used to collect samples for clotting tests, chemistry tests, physical inspection, and immunology tests.
- EDTA or heparin tubes are used for identifying the presence of crystals, performing cell counts, and preparing the sample for a smear.

- **Bone marrow** is found in the center of the bones.
  - A physician obtains a bone marrow sample by performing a needle aspiration.
  - Bone marrow tests can be used to diagnose blood and bone cancers, genetic abnormalities, and infections in the bone (osteomyelitis).
  - A phlebotomist can assist in the procedure by creating and labeling slides, or by placing the aspirated material into a culture medium, a fixative, or EDTA tubes.

- **Sputum** is mucus from the respiratory tract.
  - Sputum is used to test for infections, particularly for the bacterium that causes tuberculosis (TB).
  - The patient should cough deeply to produce the mucus and expel it into the collection tube.
  - An **acid-fast bacillus (AFB)** culture and smear are done using sputum to test for TB.

HELPFUL HINT

Special Considerations for Sputum Collection:

Patients should rinse their mouths with water before providing a sample.

Patients should give the sample first thing in the morning.

Patients should wait an hour after eating before providing a sputum specimen to avoid vomiting.

QUICK REVIEW QUESTIONS

7. Why is it important for a CSF specimen to be delivered to the laboratory for immediate testing?

8. What types of tubes might be used to store pericardial fluid samples?

Answer Key

1. A patient should wait at least 8 hours after eating before providing a fasting urine sample.

2. The patient should void into the toilet before setting the timer so that their bladder is empty when the timer starts. They will start collecting urine for the sample the next time they need to urinate.

3. Contamination by urine or blood (e.g., from hemorrhoids) can lead to an inaccurate result, as can NSAIDs, steroids, or vitamin C. Patients also need to avoid eating red meat, broccoli, cauliflower, turnips, radishes, and melons, among other foods, to avoid an inaccurate result.

4. A C-urea breath test indicates the presence of H. pylori, the bacterium believed to cause stomach ulcers.

5. DNA collection is done with a buccal (oral) swab.

6. The physician will likely order an oral hormone test. The phlebotomist will need to collect an oral fluid (saliva) sample.

7. A lumbar puncture is a painful medical procedure with possible serious side effects. Testing the sample immediately ensures that the patient will not need to undergo the procedure again.

8. Pericardial fluid is serous fluid from around the heart. Tubes that might be used include sterile tubes (for cultures), heparin or sodium fluoride tubes (for chemistry tests), nonanticoagulant tubes (for biochemical tests), and EDTA tubes (for cell counts or smears).

FOUR: SPECIMEN HANDLING, TRANSPORT, and PROCESSING

Requisition Orders

- Before a laboratory specimen is collected and tested, the provider must enter a **requisition order.**

- A lab requisition order is considered a legal document and is part of the patient's medical record.

- This requisition form may be created manually (usually on a specialized form) or on a computer system.

- The requisition order must note:
  - physician's name
  - patient's name
  - patient's medical record number
  - patient's date of birth
  - date and type of test
  - billing code
  - patient-specific precautions (e.g., fall risk)
  - test status (e.g., fasting)

- After the phlebotomist receives a lab requisition order, they must:
  1. Review the order to ensure it contains all necessary information.
  2. Verify the type of test to be performed and the conditions of the test.
  3. Verify the date and time the test is to be performed.
  4. Record the receipt of the requisition and assign it an accession number (see below) if it does not already have one.

QUICK REVIEW QUESTION

1. A phlebotomist comes to a patient's room to draw a blood specimen. While confirming the patient's ID, the phlebotomist finds that the medical records number (MRN) on the requisition form does not match the MRN on the patient's ID bracelet. What should the phlebotomist do next?

Accessioning and Labeling

- **Accessioning** is the process of recording that a test request or specimen has been received and assigning it a number for tracking purposes.
  - When a test request or specimen is accessioned, it is assigned an **accession number.**
  - Numbers may be assigned manually or by a computerized system. In a computerized system, it happens as soon as the order is entered into the system.
  - Once an accession number is assigned, all the material used to label collected specimens and track tests is grouped together by the accession number.
- **Labels** can be created manually or by a computerized system.
- Computerized systems usually create patient labels with a **bar code** that contains the patient and test information.
  - When using a computerized system with bar codes, the phlebotomist can scan a patient's wristband, match the order to the patient, and print the appropriate specimen labels at the bedside.
  - The phlebotomist's initials and the collection date and time may be hand-written on the label by the phlebotomist at the time of collection.

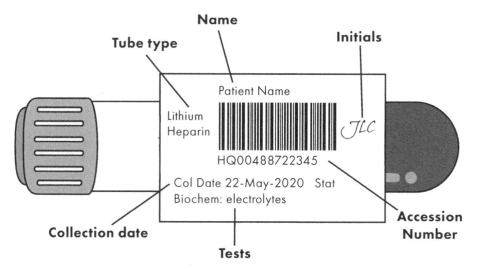

Figure 4.1. Venipuncture Label with Bar Code

- Paper requisition forms may have bar code stickers that can be attached to the sample to enable tracking.
- If the label is being created manually, document the following on all specimen labels:
  1. patient's full name with middle initial if available
  2. patient's identification number, hospital room, and bed number (if applicable)
  3. patient's date of birth
  4. date and time of collection

5. phlebotomist's name or ID number

6. special circumstances (e.g., timed test 5 minutes)

- Specimens must be labeled meticulously to avoid having specimens discarded or having results misreported.

  ○ Label the specimen in front of the patient immediately after the sample is collected.

  ○ Do not turn away from the patient before attaching the label.

  ○ Review the patient identifying information or ask the patient to look at the label and verify the information before anyone leaves the room.

  ○ Place the label on the body of the container, not on the removable cap.

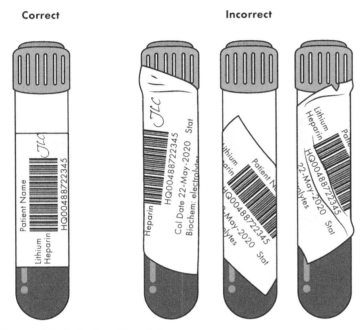

Figure 4.2. Labeling Vacutainers

QUICK REVIEW QUESTION

2. What information will a phlebotomist likely need to add to a printed specimen label once a collection is complete?

Transporting Specimens

- Blood specimens should be transported in a labeled **biohazard bag** with a liquid-tight closure.

- Specimen bags should have a storage area for related paperwork (e.g., requisition forms).

- Non-blood specimens should be transported in a sealed, secure container with a leakproof cover.

- Some specimens are transported to an **on-site laboratory**.

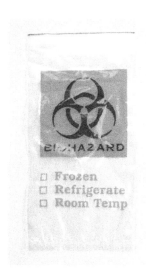

Figure 4.3. Biohazard Specimen Bag

- o Delivery may be done by hand or through an automated system.
- o Some facilities use a pneumatic tube system for the automated transport of specimens.
- o Specimens that might be affected by the destruction of blood cells or that need to be kept at body temperature cannot be transported through an automated system and must be transported by hand.
- Specimens are transported to **local offsite laboratories** via courier.
  - o The leakproof bag or container is put in a bag, box, or cooler that has a lining of absorbent material.
  - o The transport container must be properly labeled and contain identifying paperwork for each specimen.
  - o The transport container must be kept closed during transport.
  - o The transport container should be kept on the floor of the transport vehicle or secured to a seat and protected from exposure to light and air vents.
  - o Vehicles used to transport samples to a lab can only be used for that purpose.
- Time limits for testing should be considered when specimens are transported.
  - o Most routine blood samples are tested within 2 hours. Blood samples should be centrifuged before the samples are transported if tests will not be performed within 2 hours.
  - o Blood samples in gel tubes can be stored for 48 hours unless they are being tested for a substance that may be absorbed by the gel.
  - o **Stat** or **emergency orders** must be transported and tested immediately.

Table 4.1. Timing Considerations for Specimen Transport

Specimen	Timing Considerations
Ammonia	must be cooled immediately and tested within 15 minutes
EDTA blood smears	should be prepared within 1 hour of collection
EDTA specimens	should be tested within 6 hours but can be stored for up to 24 hours if refrigerated
Glucose in NaF	can be kept for 24 hours at room temperature and 48 hours if refrigerated
Glucose (pediatric)	should be tested as soon as possible
Heparin monitoring (PTT)	must be centrifuged within 1 hour and tested within 4 hours
Homocysteine (Hcy)	must be centrifuged and separated within 2 hours
Lactic acid	must be centrifuged and separated within 15 minutes
PT and PTT	can be stored for up to 24 hours but is usually tested within 4 hours
Urine	should be transported and tested promptly

- Some specimens must be kept at specific temperatures for storage and transport to prevent degradation of the specimen.

Table 4.2. Temperature Requirements for Specimens

Term	Temperature Range	Common Specimens
Body temperature	97.52°F – 99.68°F (36.4°C – 37.6°C)	cold agglutinin, cryofibrinogen, cryoglobulins
Room temperature	59°F – 86°F (15°C – 30°C)	magnesium, phosphorus, uric acid
Chilled	kept on ice or cooling rack	ammonia, some peptide tests (e.g., C-peptide)
Refrigerated	35.6°F – 50°F (2°C – 10°C)	BMP, BUN, CMV, creatinine, HCG, lipid panel, liver panel
Frozen	<–4°F (–20°C)	separated plasma or serum frozen for storage and transport of acid phosphatase, some clotting factor tests (e.g., AT-III, fibrinogen), D-dimer, DIC panel, FSP/FDP

- Some specimens will degrade when exposed to light.
  - **Light-sensitive specimens** include bilirubin, blood for certain vitamin-level tests (e.g., carotene, folate), and urine for some tests.
  - Light-sensitive specimens can be collected in specialized amber tubes or wrapped in aluminum foil to prevent exposure of the sample.

- Specimens that are shipped must follow regulations from the Department of Transportation (DOT) and International Air Transport Association (IATA).
  - Diagnostic specimens are designated Category B.
  - Specimens must be triple packaged in the following order (from inside to outside):
    1. a watertight primary container (e.g., vacutainer) that is glass, metal, or plastic
    2. a leakproof secondary container (e.g., biohazard bag)
    3. an outer container made from wood, metal, plastic, or fiberboard
  - Cooling materials should be placed between the second and third (outer) containers.
  - The outer container must be labeled "Biological Substance Category B" and include shipping information for recipient and sender.

HELPFUL HINT

Chilled specimens should be kept in a mixture of ice and water (a slurry). Keeping specimens on solid ice will cool the specimen unevenly.

QUICK REVIEW QUESTIONS

3. A phlebotomist is collecting specimens for vitamin B1, B6, and B12 testing. What special considerations will these samples need for transport?

4. What temperature should specimens for cold agglutinin testing be kept at?

Assessing Specimen Quality

- When a specimen is delivered to the lab, it will be assessed for suitability for testing.

- Possible reasons for specimen rejection include:
  - temperature or light requirements not met
  - quantity not sufficient (QNS)
  - incorrect or outdated tube
  - incorrect timing of collection or processing
  - under- or overfilled tube
  - corruption of sample (e.g., clotting or hemolysis)
  - missing or erroneous information on label

- **Hemolysis** is the damage or destruction of red blood cells that causes hemoglobin to enter the blood plasma, making it appear pink.

- Hemolysis can be caused by:
  - rough handling of specimens (e.g., shaking additive tubes)
  - incorrect equipment (e.g., using a needle whose diameter is too small)
  - incorrect technique (e.g., pulling back the syringe plunger too fast)

- Hemolysis can cause:
  - elevated levels of potassium, ammonia, iron, magnesium, and phosphate
  - decreased levels of RBCs, troponin T, alkaline phosphatase, and glucose

- When a specimen is rejected, the laboratory should notify the appropriate provider so that another specimen can be collected.

QUICK REVIEW QUESTION

5. A phlebotomist is using a needle to collect a blood sample for a CBC. During the draw, the blood is frothing as it passes from the needle into the syringe. Why will this sample likely be rejected by the laboratory?

Specimen Processing

- **Central processing** is the area in a lab where specimens are received and prepared for testing. Specimens will typically be accessioned, evaluated for quality, sorted by department and processing requirements, and prepared for testing.

- Some specimens must be centrifuged before testing.

HELPFUL HINT

Specimens that do not to be centrifuged include hematology specimens in EDTA tubes, cultures, and non-blood fluids.

- A **centrifuge** is a machine used to quickly separate blood products and other specimens by spinning them at a high number of **revolutions per minute (rpm)**.
  - The force created by the centrifuge pulls the heavier components of the specimen to the bottom of the tube.

- The force applied by the centrifuge can be measured as **relative centrifugal force (RCF)** or **gravities (g)**.
- Most samples can be centrifuged for 1.0 minutes at 1000 g. However, some samples require specific, precise force or timing.

- Pre-centrifugation considerations:
  - Plasma specimens in tubes with anticoagulants may be centrifuged immediately.
  - Serum tests cannot be centrifuged until the clotting process is complete (usually 30 minutes to 1 hour).
  - Cold samples may take longer to clot.
  - Before centrifugation, tubes should be kept in an upright position with stoppers on to prevent damage to the specimen.

- Guidelines for using a centrifuge:
  - Stoppers should be on the tubes when specimens are placed in a centrifuge.
  - Specimens that are required to be kept cold should be centrifuged in a refrigerated centrifuge.
  - Always **balance** the centrifuge, meaning distribute the tubes equally around the center.

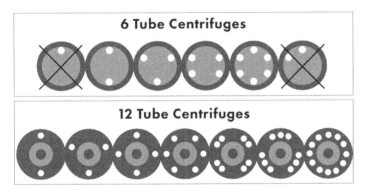

Figure 4.4. Balancing a Centrifuge

  - The lid of the centrifuge should remain closed when it is in use.
  - Do not centrifuge a specimen more than once.

- Post-centrifugation considerations:
  - If the plasma or serum contains RBCs or is pink, the specimen is invalid. A pinkish color is an indication of hemolysis.
  - Plasma and serum should be extracted from the tube as soon as possible.
  - Most plasma and serum in gel tubes can be refrigerated for up to 48 hours.
  - Plasma or serum may be removed through the stopper (i.e., with the stopper on) or with the stopper off, depending on the type of tube.
  - To remove plasma from the tube, aspirate the plasma using a syringe or pipette without touching the blood clot or cells.

HELPFUL HINT

Specimens should be thawed at room temperature. After thawing, they should be mixed by inverting ten times.

DID YOU KNOW?

Any time a verbal report is given, a written report must also be sent.

HELPFUL HINT

A *critical (panic) value* is a lab result that suggests a life-threatening condition that needs to be addressed by the provider immediately.

- An **aliquot** is a part of a larger sample that is extracted for testing.
  - Aliquots are used when one sample will be used for multiple tests.
  - To create an aliquot, use a disposable pipette to transfer plasma or serum to the aliquot tube and cap it immediately.
  - Aliquots should be carefully labeled with the same information as the original specimen.
  - Do not pour directly from the tube or "pop" the stopper—these increase the risk of exposing the phlebotomist or lab personnel to **aerosol** (a fine mist of fluid suspended in the air).
  - Specimens from tubes with different additives should never be placed in the same aliquot tube.
  - Aliquot samples can be stored for 8 hours at room temperature, refrigerated for up to 48 hours, or frozen for up to 2 weeks.
- Test results may be reported in several different ways:
  - automatically through a computerized system that connects the laboratory to the patient's electronic medical record
  - printed and delivered to the appropriate personnel
  - delivered via phone (more common for stat or emergency testing)
- The phlebotomist's role in reporting lab results includes:
  - verifying that an electronic report is accurate
  - ensuring that printed lab reports are distributed appropriately
  - calling or paging a provider with the results of a stat or emergency lab test
  - recognizing critical values and reporting them appropriately

QUICK REVIEW QUESTIONS

6. A phlebotomist has collected a green plasma separator tube (PST) and a red serum tube. Which of these tubes can be centrifuged first?

7. Why should blood specimens be stored upright with the stopper up?

Point-of-Care Testing

- **Point-of-care testing** (**POCT**) is done near the patient, not in a laboratory.
  - POCT has a quick turnaround time and is more convenient for the patient and provider.
  - Point-of-care tests are waived tests, meaning they are simple to perform and have a low risk of error.
- The chemical component of urinalysis can be done at point of care using a urine **dipstick** that is placed in a urine sample.
  - The reagent pads on the dipstick change color when components being tested for are present.
  - The dipstick can be read by comparing it to the color chart provided by the manufacturer. Some dipsticks may be read by machines called reflectance photometers.

Table 4.3. Urinalysis Dipstick Testing

Testing for	Purpose	Normal Reading or Range
Leukocytes	Presence of WBCs indicates infection.	negative
Nitrate	Nitrates indicate infection by gram-negative bacteria.	negative
Urobilinogen	Urobilinogen indicates liver disease.	0.2 – 1 mg
Protein	Protein may indicate kidney disease or eclampsia.	negative
pH	Decreased (acidic) pH may indicate systemic acidosis or diabetes mellitus; increased (alkali) pH may indicate systemic alkalosis or UTI.	4.5 – 8
Blood	Blood in urine may indicate infection, kidney stones, or coagulation disorders.	negative
Specific gravity	This measures the concentration of urine, which can be affected by kidney or metabolic disorders.	1.010 – 1.025
Ketone	Ketones are produced during fat metabolism; their presence may indicate diabetes, hyperglycemia, starvation, alcoholism, or eclampsia.	negative
Bilirubin	Bilirubin is produced during the breakdown of heme; its presence may indicate liver disease.	negative
Glucose	Glucose in urine indicates hyperglycemia.	0 – 15 mg/dL

- Glucose levels in the blood can be tested at the point of care with small, portable glucose meters.
    - A small amount of blood from a skin puncture is placed on the test strip, and the meter provides a readout of the glucose level.
    - Glucose meters should be quality-control tested regularly (usually every 24 hours) using low and high control solutions provided by the manufacturer.
    - Normal blood glucose levels are 70 – 100 mg/dL.
- Point-of-care coagulation testing may include PT, INR, PTT, aPTT, or ACT.
    - POC coagulation testing is performed on patients taking anticoagulants (e.g., heparin, warfarin) and to assess patients before surgery.
    - PT/INR testing is done for patients taking warfarin and requires a fingerstick.
    - ACT testing is done for patients taking heparin. Most systems for POC ACT testing include a cartridge to be filled with fresh, whole blood.

QUICK REVIEW QUESTION

8. What is the purpose of low and high test control solutions for glucose meters?

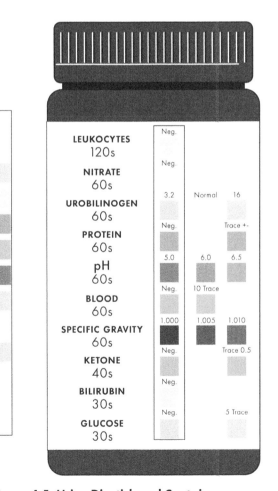

Figure 4.5. Urine Dipstick and Container

Answer Key

1. The phlebotomist should alert the nurse or other provider that the MRN on the requisition form does not match the patient's ID bracelet. The phlebotomist should not perform the blood draw until the discrepancy has been resolved and they have a requisition form that matches the patient's ID bracelet.

2. The phlebotomist will need to write the date and time of collection on the label and should initial or sign the label. They may also need to add notes specific to the testing conditions (e.g., "non-fasting").

3. Most vitamin-test specimens, including those for B vitamins, are light sensitive. The specimens should be stored and transported in amber tubes or wrapped in aluminum foil.

4. Cold agglutinin specimens should be placed on a warming device and maintained at body temperature (36.4°C – 37.6°C) immediately after collection and allowed to clot. They may be stored at room temperature after clotting is complete.

5. Frothing in the blood sample will destroy red blood cells, causing hemolysis. Because a CBC measures red blood cell levels, hemolyzed samples cannot be used.

6. The PST can be centrifuged immediately. The serum tube cannot be centrifuged until clotting is complete, which usually takes at least 30 minutes.

7. Storing blood specimens with the stopper up keeps blood away from the stopper, which helps prevent aerosol spray when the tube is opened. Transporting the tube vertically also helps prevent hemolysis caused by the blood moving in the tube.

8. Test control solutions are provided by the manufacturers of glucose meters so they can be quality-control checked. The low solution (for low glucose levels) and high solution (for high glucose levels) should each be applied to separate test strips. If the meter is working properly, it will give the value provided by the manufacturer for each solution. If the meter gives values outside the test ranges, it should not be used.

FIVE: LABORATORY OPERATIONS

Important Legislation

- The **Clinical Laboratory Improvement Amendments (CLIA)** statute was passed by Congress in 1988 to improve the quality of laboratory testing.
  - Under this legislation, all laboratories must follow certain quality control and quality assurance standards. (See "Quality Assurance and Control" below.)
  - Quality assurance does not apply to CLIA **waived tests**, which CLIA has determined are easy to perform and have a low risk of error.
  - Tests that are designated by CLIA as moderate or high complexity must be performed by qualified laboratory technicians.

Table 5.1. CLIA Test Classifications

Category	Examples
waived	urinalysis, dipstick, fecal occult blood (guaiac), urine pregnancy test, blood glucose, hemoglobin and hematocrit, erythrocyte sedimentation rate (ESR), strep A test
moderate-complexity tests	blood chemistry performed with automated analyzer, hematology performed with automated analyzer, gram staining, microscopic analysis of urine
high-complexity tests	cytology testing, blood crossmatching, blood typing, Pap smears

- In 1996, the United States federal government enacted the **Health Insurance Portability and Accountability Act (HIPAA)**, which governs the security and protection of electronic medical records (EMR) and electronic health records (EHR).
  - **Protected health information (PHI)** is any health information that can be linked to a specific individual.

○ In most cases, an authorization form signed by the patient is required before the release of any PHI.

○ HIPAA allows for the disclosure of PHI without a signed authorization form when that information will be used for treatment, payment, or health care operations.

- The **Americans with Disabilities Act Amendments Act (ADAAA)** was originally passed in 1990 as the **Americans with Disabilities Act (ADA)**.
  ○ The ADAAA, which went into effect January 1, 2009, made substantial changes to and broadened the scope of the ADA's definition of a disability.
  ○ The ADA prohibits employers with more than fifteen employees from discriminating against individuals with disabilities.
  ○ The ADA also provides protection for those seeking medical services. Patients with disabilities must be given the same opportunities to receive the same level of care as those without disabilities.

- The **Patient Protection and Affordable Care Act (ACA)** (colloquially referred to as "Obamacare") is a federal statute signed into law in 2010. Key components of the ACA include:
  ○ eliminating the ability for insurance companies to deny coverage due to a preexisting condition
  ○ prohibiting insurance companies from charging more for preexisting conditions or specific genders
  ○ allowing adults to remain on their parents' policies until the age of 26
  ○ requiring that all health care plans cover essential health benefits
  ○ eliminating annual spending caps on essential health benefits

- The **Needlestick Safety and Prevention Act** was passed in 2001. The act required OSHA to update standards for needlestick safety technology and procedures.

QUICK REVIEW QUESTION

1. Under what circumstances can a phlebotomist share PHI?

Regulatory Agencies

- The **Occupational Safety and Health Administration (OSHA)** is a federal agency under the US Department of Labor.
  ○ OSHA sets and enforces workplace standards to prevent on-the-job injuries and protect American workers.
  ○ OSHA standards regulate workplace procedures related to blood-borne pathogens (discussed in more detail in "Infection and Exposure Control," below).

- The **Centers for Disease Control and Prevention (CDC)** is an agency of the federal government within the Department of Health and Human Services.

- The main goals of the CDC are to protect and improve public health and safety through research and collaboration.
  - The CDC publishes multiple resources to assist health care providers with assessing and reducing exposure to infectious disease in the workplace.
- The **Clinical and Laboratory Standards Institute (CLSI)** is a nonprofit organization that develops standards for clinical and laboratory practices.
- The **National Accrediting Agency for Clinical Laboratory Sciences (NAACLS)** is a nonprofit organization that provides accreditation to education programs, including phlebotomy programs.
- The **American Society for Clinical Pathology (ASCP)** is a nonprofit organization for laboratory professionals.
- The **College of American Pathologists (CAP)** provides accreditation for laboratories.
- The **Joint Commission (TJC)** is a nonprofit organization that sets standards and provides accreditation for the majority of hospital and medical services in the US.
- The **Centers for Medicare and Medicaid Services (CMS)** is a federal agency within the US Department of Health and Human Services.
  - CMS administers the Medicare and Medicaid programs.
  - CMS also develops and enforces regulatory standards related to HIPAA and CLIA.

DID YOU KNOW?
Accreditation is the process of certifying that an organization meets a specific set of standards.

QUICK REVIEW QUESTION

2. How do standards set by the Occupational Safety and Health Administration (OSHA) impact the work environment of a phlebotomist?

Legal Terms

- **Criminal law** regulates behavior that is considered an offense against society, such as theft or assault.
  - Charges are issued against a person by the government, and the outcome of a trial is usually decided by a jury.
  - The most serious criminal violations are **felonies**, which are punishable by fines or prison sentences in excess of one year.
  - **Misdemeanors** are less serious crimes punishable by probation or short jail sentences.
- **Civil law** regulates behavior between individuals or individual entities. Civil law includes contracts and torts.
  - **Contract laws** involve the rights and obligations of contracts, which are binding agreements between two or more parties.
  - A **tort** is a wrongful civil act. Tort laws deal with the accidental or intentional harm to a person or property that results from the wrongdoing of a person or persons.

- **Negligence** is a type of tort. It is the failure to offer an acceptable standard of care that is comparable to what a competent medical assistant, nurse, or other health care worker would provide in a similar situation. There are four types of negligence:
  - nonfeasance: a willful failure to act when required
  - misfeasance: a willful incorrect or improper performance of a lawful action
  - malfeasance: a willful and intentional action that causes harm
  - **malpractice**: a professional's failure to properly execute their duties

QUICK REVIEW QUESTION

3. During a routine venipuncture in the antecubital fossa region, the patient complains of intense, shooting pain down to their hand when the needle is inserted. The phlebotomist says the draw will be quick and finishes collecting the specimen. The patient later develops complex regional pain syndrome due to nerve damage. What type of tort can the phlebotomist face legal action for?

Quality Assurance and Control

- **Quality assurance (QA)** is a set of protocols designed to prevent errors.
  - The goal of health care QA programs is to identify how errors occur and make corrections to procedures to prevent future problems.
  - Laboratory QA programs follow standards set by outside organizations such as TJC and CLIA.
  - QA programs are designed and implemented by management-level staff in clinical laboratories, hospitals, and other health care provider settings.

- **Quality control (QC)** is the standardized use of checks to ensure that procedures are performed without error.

- QC is performed by phlebotomists and other laboratory technicians. Examples of QC measures include:
  - using two or more identifiers to ID patients
  - inspecting equipment before procedures for damage or expiration
  - including all necessary information on specimen labels
  - filling out inspection logs after equipment inspection
  - regularly calibrating testing equipment
  - regularly monitoring temperature of storage facilities
  - completing **incident reports** when injuries occur
  - completing a **near miss** or **occurrence report** when errors occur

QUICK REVIEW QUESTION

4. A phlebotomist enters a patient's room in a hospital to draw a specimen for cardiac biomarkers. The patient is conscious and alert. The phlebotomist scans the bar code on the patient's wrist and prints labels. They perform the draw and then attach the labels to the specimens. What quality control check did the phlebotomist not perform?

Interpersonal Communication

- **Communication** is an essential part of a phlebotomist's day-to-day work as they interact with patients, their families, and other health care professionals.

- **Verbal communication** refers to words that are spoken or written.
  - ○ Verbal communication style should be appropriate for the situation.
  - ○ Avoid using abbreviated names, technical jargon, or complex medical terminology with patients.
  - ○ Use accurate technical language with other health care professionals.
  - ○ Speak at a normal volume and use a professional tone when speaking with patients and other staff.

- **Nonverbal communication** includes all the physical aspects of communication, including posture, facial expression, and eye contact. Nonverbal communication guidelines include:
  - ○ maintaining good posture (e.g., not slouching on a desk)
  - ○ keeping a polite facial expression when dealing with patients and the health care team
  - ○ respecting other people's personal boundaries (e.g., not hugging coworkers or touching patients without their consent)
  - ○ maintaining eye contact when speaking with patients and the health care team (but recognizing that there are cultural differences regarding what is appropriate)
  - ○ not using rude or inappropriate hand gestures (but keeping in mind cultural differences)

- **Active listening** means paying complete attention to the speaker, not just hearing their words. The active listener should:
  - ○ make eye contact with the speaker to indicate interest in what is being said
  - ○ not interrupt the speaker
  - ○ repeat important points the speaker has made to ensure understanding
  - ○ ask follow-up questions

- Phlebotomists will often encounter members of certain populations who may require specialized communication techniques. These groups are summarized in Table 5.1.

Table 5.1. Communicating with Diverse Populations

Population	Communication Techniques
Blind or low vision	Announce when you enter or leave the room.
	Address the patient by name.
	Describe the layout of the room.
	Narrate your actions.

Table 5.1. Communicating with Diverse Populations (continued)

Population	Communication Techniques
Deaf or hard of hearing	Speak slowly and clearly but naturally. Face the patient while you speak. Provide written materials. Use a sign language interpreter when needed.
Geriatric	Adjust language for confused or cognitively impaired patients. Rely on family members or caregivers as needed.
Pediatric	Move to patient's eye level. Use simple language. Explain exam procedures before you start. Allow patient to hold blunt, safe instruments.
Intellectually disabled	Match the patient's level of vocabulary and sentence complexity. Speak directly to the patient.
Non-reading (illiterate)	Notice when patients do not read materials. Read or explain important documents.
Non-English speaking	Have materials available in multiple languages. Use an interpreter when needed.
Anxious, angry, or distraught	Stay calm and speak clearly. Wait for the patient to calm down before relaying complex information.
Socially, culturally, or ethnically diverse	Understand that many aspects of communication, including voice volume and eye contact, have a cultural component. Be respectful of the cultural needs of patients.

QUICK REVIEW QUESTION

5. After greeting a patient and confirming the patient's ID, a phlebotomist reviews the test requisition form while the client is explaining the reason for their visit. How does this interaction show poor communication skills?

Ethics

- **Ethics** are moral principles, values, and duties set either formally or informally by peers, the community, and professional organizations.

- Various professional organizations have codes of ethics applicable to the phlebotomist, including the American Medical Association (AMA), the American Hospital Association (AHA), and the American Society for Clinical Laboratory Science (ASCLS).

- The ASCLS code of ethics includes the following principles the phlebotomist is expected to follow:
  - placing patients' welfare above their own needs and desires
  - ensuring that each patient receives care that is safe, effective, efficient, timely, equitable, and patient-centered
  - maintaining dignity and respect for the profession
  - promoting the advancement of the profession
  - ensuring collegial relationships within the clinical laboratory and with other patient care providers
  - improving access to laboratory services
  - promoting equitable distribution of health care resources
  - complying with laws and regulations and protecting patients from others' incompetent or illegal practice
  - changing conditions when necessary to advance the best interests of patients
- Phlebotomists have an ethical duty to act within their **scope of practice**—the procedures they are trained and licensed to perform.
- The phlebotomist's scope of practice includes:
  - collecting blood via venipuncture and capillary puncture
  - transporting and processing specimens
  - performing some waived and point-of-care tests
- A phlebotomist may not do any of the following:
  - make medical diagnoses
  - administer medications
  - start IVs
  - perform non-waived tests
  - perform certain types of specimen collection (e.g., cerebrospinal fluid, blood from an IV)

QUICK REVIEW QUESTION

6. What kind of specimens can a phlebotomist collect when acting within their scope of practice?

Infection and Exposure Control

- The goal of **infection control** is to intervene in the chain of infection at the point where infection is most likely to occur in order to prevent its spread.
- When an organism establishes an opportunistic relationship with a host, the process is called **infection**.
- Infections can be caused by many different infectious agents.
  - **Bacteria** are single-celled prokaryotic organisms that are responsible for many common infections such as strep throat, urinary tract infections, and many food-borne illnesses.

- **Viruses** are composed of a nucleic acid (DNA or RNA) wrapped in a protein capsid. Viral infections include the common cold, influenza, and human immunodeficiency virus (HIV).
- **Protozoa** are single-celled eukaryotic organisms. Protozoan infections include giardia (an intestinal infection) and African sleeping sickness.
- **Fungi** are a group of eukaryotic organisms that include yeasts, molds, and mushrooms. Common fungal infections are athlete's foot, ringworm, and oral and vaginal yeast infections.
- Parasitic diseases are caused by **parasites** that live in or on the human body and use its resources. Common human parasites include worms (e.g., tapeworms), flukes, lice, and ticks.

- Infections travel from person to person via the **chain of infection**.
  - The chain starts with a **causative organism** (e.g., a bacteria or virus).
  - The organism needs a **reservoir**, or place to live. This may be biological, such as people or animals, or it may be environmental (e.g., surface of a table).
  - In order to spread, the infectious agent needs a way to **exit** the reservoir, such as being expelled as droplets during a sneeze.
  - For the infection chain to continue, the infectious agent needs to encounter a susceptible **host**—a person who can become infected.
  - Finally, the infectious agent needs a way to **enter** the host, such as through inhalation or drinking contaminated water.

- There are a variety of modes of transmission for infectious agents.
  - **Direct contact** is transmission from one infected person to another during physical contact with blood or other body fluids (e.g., transmission of herpes during sexual intercourse).
  - **Indirect contact** is transmission of the disease through a nonbiological reservoir (e.g., drinking water contaminated with giardia).
  - **Droplets** are infectious agents trapped in moisture that are expelled when an infected person sneezes or coughs. They can enter the respiratory system of other people and cause infection (e.g., transmission of influenza when an infected person sneezes).
  - Some droplets are light enough to remain airborne, meaning people may inhale infectious agents from the air long after the initial cough or sneeze (e.g., measles, which can live in airborne droplets for up to two hours).
  - Some diseases are carried by organisms called **vectors** that spread the disease; the infection does not require direct physical contact between people (e.g., mosquitoes carrying malaria).

- **Personal protective equipment (PPE)** is any item necessary for the prevention of microorganism transmission. PPE includes gloves, gowns, goggles, eye shields, and masks.
- **Standard precautions** (also called universal precautions) are based on the assumption that all patients are infected with microorganisms. Standard precautions should be used when the provider may contact body fluids (except sweat), non-intact skin, or mucous membranes. *Always all the time*
  - Practice appropriate hand hygiene.

○ Use PPE.

○ Prevent needlesticks and sharps injuries.

○ Clean and disinfect equipment and environmental surfaces.

○ Follow respiratory hygiene guidelines (cough etiquette).

○ Dispose of waste properly.

○ Follow all protocols for safe, sterile injections.

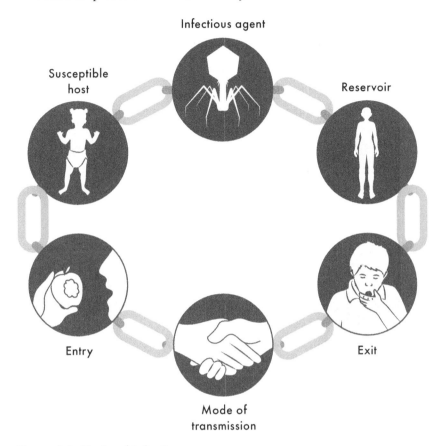

Figure 5.1. Chain of Infection

- Additional precautions may be needed for patients with known infections. These precautions are based on the transmission route for the infection.

  ○ **Airborne precautions** require the use of N-95 respirator masks and negative-pressure air systems.

  ○ **Droplet precautions** require the use of appropriate PPE and washing hands thoroughly after removing gloves.

  ○ **Contact precautions** require appropriate PPE, removing PPE immediately after leaving the patient, and disinfecting common equipment after use.

- **Regulated medical waste (RMW)** (also called biohazardous waste) is any waste that is or may be contaminated with infectious materials, including blood, secretions, and excretions.

  ○ **Sharps** should be disposed of in a biohazard sharps container. The term "sharps" refers to needles, lancets, blood tubes, capillary tubes, razor blades, suturing needles, hypodermic needles, and microscope slides and coverslips.

- Blood and body fluids, such as urine, sputum, semen, amniotic fluid, and cerebrospinal fluid, can be disposed of in a drain, toilet, or utility sink.
  - Feces should be flushed in a toilet.
  - Bandages, dressing gauzes, and gloves with small amounts of RMW can be put in regular garbage disposal cans.
  - Dirty linen should be put in a separate receptacle; if very soiled by blood, it should be put in a biohazard bag.
- **Asepsis** is the absence of infectious organisms.
  - An object that has had all infectious agents removed or destroyed is **sterile**.
  - **Medical asepsis** is the practice of destroying infectious agents outside the body to prevent the spread of disease.
  - Medical asepsis is different from **clean technique**, which also aims to minimize the spread of infectious agents but does not require sterilization. Wearing gloves is an example of clean technique: the gloves are not sterile, but they provide a barrier that prevents the spread of infection from patient to provider.
  - **Surgical asepsis** is the practice of removing all infectious pathogens from all equipment involved in invasive procedures.

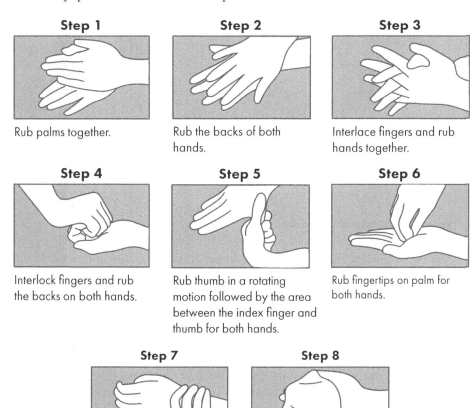

Step 1
Rub palms together.

Step 2
Rub the backs of both hands.

Step 3
Interlace fingers and rub hands together.

Step 4
Interlock fingers and rub the backs on both hands.

Step 5
Rub thumb in a rotating motion followed by the area between the index finger and thumb for both hands.

Step 6
Rub fingertips on palm for both hands.

Step 7
Rub both wrists in a rotating motion.

Step 8
Rinse and dry thoroughly.

Figure 5.2. Aseptic Handwashing Technique

- ○ **Aseptic handwashing** is a specific technique intended to remove all infectious agents from the hands and wrists.
- **Blood-borne pathogens** are microorganisms found in human blood and tissue.
- Blood-borne pathogens that pose a risk for phlebotomists include:
  - ○ human immunodeficiency virus (HIV), a virus that attacks the immune system
  - ○ hepatitis B (HBV), hepatitis C (HCV), and hepatitis D (HDV), viruses that attack the liver
  - ○ cytomegalovirus, a common virus that usually has no symptoms but may lead to more serious disorders in people with compromised immune systems
- OSHA maintains standards for universal precautions against blood-borne pathogens, and employers may face penalties if these protocols are not followed. According to the standards, employers must provide:
  - ○ all necessary PPE
  - ○ environmental control methods, including access to clean air and water and appropriate processes for waste disposal
  - ○ training on blood-borne pathogens for employees
  - ○ an **exposure control plan** that explains steps to be taken by employees exposed to blood-borne pathogens
- Exposure to blood-borne pathogens requires immediate action.
  - ○ For a needlestick, remove object from wound and clean the site with soap and water.
  - ○ For membrane exposure (splashes), flush site with water or saline for 10 minutes.
- Spills of body fluids or chemicals should be cleaned up as soon as possible with **spill kits**.
  - ○ Kits may contain specialized materials for cleaning specific substances.
  - ○ Always wear gloves when cleaning spills.
  - ○ Disinfect spill area with an EPA-approved disinfectant.
- Although rare, **fires** can occur in health care offices. The phlebotomist should cooperate with the following fire safety measures:
  - ○ keeping open spaces free of clutter
  - ○ marking fire exits
  - ○ knowing the locations of fire exits, alarms, and extinguishers
  - ○ knowing the fire drill and evacuation plan of the health care facility
  - ○ not using the elevator when a fire occurs
  - ○ turning off oxygen in the vicinity of a fire
- Guidelines for **electrical safety** include:
  - ○ inspecting electrical equipment for defects
  - ○ discarding electrical cords that are exposed, damaged, or frayed
  - ○ never running electrical wiring under carpets
  - ○ not unplugging an item by yanking the cord

DID YOU KNOW?

Chemicals should be stored and disposed of according to the information in their **safety data sheets (SDS)**, which are provided by the manufacturer.

- never using electrical appliances near bathtubs, sinks, or other water sources
- disconnecting plugs from outlets before cleaning appliances or equipment

QUICK REVIEW QUESTION

7. A phlebotomist has been asked to collect a feces sample from a patient with a suspected *C. difficile* infection, which is spread through contact with feces. What PPE should the phlebotomist use?

Medical Emergencies

- A medical emergency is an unexpected life-threatening event. It can occur at any time, so the phlebotomist must be prepared and know what to do.

- **Cardiopulmonary (cardiac) arrest** occurs when the heart stops beating, which causes blood to stop flowing.
  - The patient will have no pulse and either will not be breathing or will display labored breathing (agonal gasps).
  - **Cardiopulmonary resuscitation (CPR)** should be started immediately for any patient in cardiac arrest.

- **Respiratory arrest** occurs when breathing stops or is no longer effective at meeting the body's oxygen needs.
  - Respiratory arrest often occurs with cardiac arrest but can occur alone as well. It will eventually lead to cardiac arrest.
  - **Rescue breathing** should be started for patients in respiratory arrest.

- When a patient is having a **seizure**, the following guidelines will help protect them:
  - Remove any objects in the area that might cause injury.
  - Loosen tight clothing.
  - Do not restrain a seizing patient.
  - Do not place anything in the patient's mouth.
  - If needed, place the patient in the recovery position (on their side).

- **Shock** occurs when the cardiovascular system is compromised.
  - **Cardiogenic shock** occurs when the heart can no longer pump effectively, reducing blood flow and available oxygen throughout the body. This type of shock is most commonly seen in individuals having a heart attack.
  - **Hypovolemic shock** (decrease in blood volume) occurs when rapid fluid loss decreases circulating blood volume and cardiac output, resulting in inadequate blood flow to tissues.
  - **Septic shock** is the result of a massive inflammatory response to systemic infection. It can lead to multi-organ failure and death.
  - Signs and symptoms of cardiogenic, hypovolemic, and septic shock are similar and may include:
    - hypotension (low blood pressure)
    - rapid heart rate

- difficulty breathing
  - cool, clammy skin
  - low urine output
- All types of shock are considered life-threatening conditions and require immediate transfer to a higher level of care.

- There are three types of bleeding: arterial, venous, and capillary.
  - **Arterial bleeding** occurs when an artery is damaged. Arterial blood is bright red and "spurts" due to the pressure of the heart pumping. The blood is often moving too quickly for clotting to occur. Arterial bleeding can be life-threatening and requires immediate intervention.
  - **Venous bleeding** occurs when a vein is damaged. Veins carry high volumes of blood, but they do not supply the same pressure as arteries, so venous bleeding is slower than arterial bleeding. The blood is also darker in color because it is deoxygenated.
  - **Capillary bleeding** occurs when the small blood vessels that create the network between veins and arteries are damaged. Capillary bleeding is often seen in wound beds or with skin abrasions. Bleeding from the capillaries is usually controlled easily.
  - The treatment for all types of bleeding is to apply direct pressure to the site.
    1. Observe standard precautions, including wearing gloves.
    2. Place the patient in a prone position.
    3. Apply pressure using sterile gauze. Pressure may be applied for up to 20 minutes depending on the type of bleed.
    4. If the bleed is arterial, pressure may be applied above the site of bleeding (only if directed by the provider).
    5. Continue to evaluate for symptoms of shock.
    6. Assist with cleaning and dressing the wound once the bleeding has stopped.

DID YOU KNOW?

Do not remove blood-soaked dressings, as this will interrupt the clotting process. Instead, add gauze as necessary.

QUICK REVIEW QUESTION

8. What signs and symptoms are seen in patients with cardiogenic shock?

Medical Coding

- A universal set of codes is used to simplify health care communication, particularly for reimbursement.

- The **International Classification of Diseases (ICD)** is a coding system used to classify diseases. The tenth revision, known as ICD-10, is currently in use.
  - Each ICD code corresponds to a different medical diagnosis.
  - The ICD-10 codes are alphanumeric. The first character is always a letter, and the second character is always a number. The rest of the code contains between one and five more characters. (For example, the ICD-10 code for fatty [change of] liver is K76.0.)

- **Current Procedural Terminology (CPT)** uses a set of standardized five-digit codes to identify medical, surgical, or diagnostic services.
  - CPT codes refer only to medical procedures and are used with ICD codes (which give the diagnosis for the underlying medical condition).
  - A **CPT code modifier (CM)** is added to a CPT code to give extra information to insurance companies.
- Every CPT code must be linked to a corresponding ICD code to support the medical necessity for the service or procedure performed. For example, an ICD diagnosis of iron deficiency anemia (D50.9) could be given as the reason for a CBC with differential, which is CPT code 85025.
- The **Healthcare Common Procedure Coding System (HCPCS)** is a set of medical codes used when filing Medicare claims. HCPCS Level I codes are the numeric CPT codes. Level II codes are alphanumeric and are usually for non-physician services (e.g., ambulance transport).
- A **diagnosis-related group (DRG)** is a classification system used to determine payments for hospitalized Medicare patients.
  - Each DRG is a three-digit number describing a specific diagnosis (e.g., 176: pulmonary embolism without MCC).
  - Medicare then determines the cost of the average resources used to treat patients in that DRG and pays the hospital a flat rate for each patient assigned that DRG.

QUICK REVIEW QUESTION

9. Which procedure code set should be used when billing Medicaid or Medicare?

Billing

- **Health insurance companies** act as the financial intermediary between patients and medical providers.
- Consumers can purchase insurance plans through their employer as part of a group plan or through the **health insurance marketplace** established under the ACA.
- The consumer pays the insurance company a **premium**—a regular, predetermined amount of money. In return, the insurer covers some amount of the financial costs of the consumer's medical care.
- In addition to the cost of their premium, patients also share the cost of their medical expenses through payments referred to as co-pays, deductibles, and coinsurance.
  - **Co-pays** are set payments that patients pay every time they seek medical care. For example, their insurance might require a fifteen-dollar co-pay every time they see their medical provider.
  - A **deductible** is a set amount that patients must pay before the insurance company will cover any of their medical care.

DID YOU KNOW?

In a PPO, providers are usually compensated using a **fee-for-service** arrangement in which they bill the insurance company for each separate service provided.

- ○ **Coinsurance** is the total percentage of the costs of a patient's medical care that an insurance company will pay.
- There are four main types of insurance programs available to patients:
  - ○ In a **preferred provider organization (PPO)**, the company has a **network** of providers, and patients pay higher rates to see providers outside the network.
  - ○ An **exclusive provider organization (EPO)** is similar to a PPO, but the insurance company will not cover any **out-of-network** services.
  - ○ In a **health maintenance organization (HMO)**, patients must get referrals from a primary care provider (PCP) for all services, and only in-network costs are covered.
  - ○ **Point-of-service (POS)** plans require patients to get referrals from a PCP, but the insurance company will cover some out-of-network costs.
- The US federal government provides health insurance for select individuals through various programs:
  - ○ **Medicare** covers health care costs for taxpayers over 65 or people under 65 with certain disabilities or disorders like end-stage renal disease.
  - ○ **Medicaid** is a joint federal-state program that provides health coverage for individuals with low incomes.
  - ○ **Social Security Disability Insurance (SSDI)** is a benefit program for people who are blind or disabled and cannot work.
  - ○ **TRICARE** is a health care program for military personnel and their families.
  - ○ **CHAMPVA** is another military health coverage benefit that provides comprehensive health coverage for a spouse or dependent of a veteran who is permanently disabled due to military service.

QUICK REVIEW QUESTION

10. Which insurance program covers people 65 or older, younger people with disabilities, and people with end-stage renal disease?

Answer Key

1. PHI can be shared when the patient has signed an authorization form allowing the release of the information. PHI that is directly relevant to care can also be shared with other providers involved in the patient's care (e.g., sending test results to a primary care provider).

2. OSHA's workplace safety standards directly impact the work environment of phlebotomists in a number of ways. OSHA's blood-borne pathogens standards require employers to provide specific training and equipment for managing exposure to blood-borne pathogens. OSHA also regulates the ways employers choose, label, and store hazardous chemicals. Many general OSHA safety standards apply to the phlebotomist's work environment, including those related to ladder use, electrical safety, and emergency exits.

3. The phlebotomist and/or their employer may be sued for malpractice. Standards of care for a phlebotomist require that they immediately withdraw the needle if the patient reports severe pain. The phlebotomist likely committed malpractice by continuing the collection.

4. The phlebotomist should always get two forms of ID before drawing a specimen, and when possible should actively involve the patient in the identification process. The phlebotomist should have asked the patient to confirm their name or DOB and checked the information on the ID bracelet against the test requisition form.

5. While the patient is speaking, the phlebotomist should show they are listening by making eye contact. They should avoid checking the form until the patient has finished speaking.

6. Phlebotomists can collect blood specimens via capillary puncture and venipuncture. They may also collect urine and feces samples; nasal, oral, or throat swabs; breath samples; and saliva samples.

7. *C. difficile* requires contact protections, so the phlebotomist should use gloves and an isolation gown.

8. Classic signs of cardiogenic shock include hypotension, a rapid pulse that weakens, cool, clammy skin, and decreased urine output.

9. The Healthcare Common Procedure Coding System (HCPCS) should be used when billing Medicaid or Medicare.

10. Medicare is the federal health insurance program that covers people sixty-five or older, younger people with disabilities, and people with end-stage renal disease.

SIX: PRACTICE TEST

DIRECTIONS: READ THE QUESTION, AND THEN CHOOSE THE MOST CORRECT ANSWER.

1. Which of the following structures begins the heartbeat by starting an electrical impulse in the right atrium?

   A) atrioventricular (AV) node

   B) sinoatrial (SA) node

   C) bundle of His

   D) mitral valve

2. Which of the following is the correct way a phlebotomist should introduce themselves to the patient?

   A) "Hi. I'm the phlebotomist, here to draw your blood tests."

   B) "Hi. I'm here to draw your lab work."

   C) "Hi. My name is Jaime Smith. I'm the phlebotomist who will be drawing your lab work this morning."

   D) "Hi. My name is Jaime. I'm here to draw your labs."

3. What are casts?

   A) bacteria in urine

   B) metabolized drug particles in urine

   C) preservatives added to a specimen cup

   D) cylindrical structures in urine

4. How many identifiers must the phlebotomist request to confirm a patient's identity before drawing blood?

   A) 1

   B) 2

   C) 3

   D) 4

5. What is important to do when communicating with an anxious or angry patient?

   A) provide patient education

   B) call security

   C) stay calm and speak clearly, using short and simple sentences

   D) tell them you will come back when they are calm

6. Which of the following should NOT be used to confirm the identity of a patient before venipuncture?

   A) date of birth

   B) Social Security number

   C) medical record number

   D) room number

7. Which of the following arteries carries deoxygenated blood? *to lung*

   A) aorta

   B) pulmonary artery

   C) radial artery

   D) femoral artery

8. An unconscious patient is brought to the emergency department with no identification. How should the phlebotomist ensure that the patient's samples are labeled correctly?

   A) do not draw samples until the patient is awake and can confirm their identity

   B) look in the patient's wallet for identification

   C) use the temporary name and number assigned to the patient

   D) label the sample with the room number and mental status of the patient

9. What is a requisition order?

   A) a doctor's written instructions

   B) the laboratory supply list

   C) a phlebotomist's list of specimen collections for the day

   D) the order in which specimens need to be collected

10. While verifying a patient's identity, the phlebotomist notes that the date of birth on the patient's wristband is incorrect. What is the next step?

   A) proceed after the patient verbally states their correct date of birth

   B) cross it out with a permanent marker and initial the change

   C) do not proceed until the discrepancy is corrected

   D) alert a nurse and have them note the error in the patient's chart

11. A 19-year-old, nonverbal, mentally impaired patient in the ICU has morning blood work ordered by their doctor. Which of the following is NOT an acceptable way to confirm that the patient's identity matches the information on the wristband ID?

   A) ask the patient to signal their verification by nodding *Don't do this*

   B) verify the patient's name and date of birth with the nurse

   C) verify the patient's name and date of birth with a parent or guardian who is sitting at the bedside

   D) verify the patient's name and date of birth with the physician

12. Gas exchange occurs in which type of blood vessel?

   A) venule

   B) vein

   C) capillary

   D) arteriole

13. Which of the following are symptoms of shock?

   A) low blood pressure and clammy skin

   B) increased urine output and shortness of breath

   C) nausea and vomiting with pain in the abdomen

   D) high blood pressure and warm skin

14. When is a postprandial test done?

   A) 2 hours before eating a meal

   B) 1 hour after waking

   C) 2 hours after exercise

   D) 2 hours after eating a meal

15. A laboratory has a set of samples that include ASAP, fasting, timed, and routine specimens. Which specimens should be processed first?

    A) ASAP *STAT*

    B) fasting

    C) timed

    D) routine

16. What happens during accessioning?

    A) The specimens are labeled with the patient's name.

    B) Numbers are assigned to specimens for tracking purposes.

    C) The order is given to staff to complete.

    D) Samples are balanced in a centrifuge.

17. "Basal state" refers to the body's metabolic state:

    A) after fasting for 12 hours

    B) 2 hours after a meal

    C) immediately after glucose ingestion

    D) while asleep

18. What is used to obtain a urine sample from an infant?

    A) urinary catheter

    B) toilet hat

    C) urinary collection bag

    D) commode

19. The set of standardized five-digit codes used to identify medical, surgical, or diagnostic services is called:

    A) Diagnosis-Related Group

    B) Current Procedural Terminology

    C) International Classification of Diseases

    D) Healthcare Common Procedure Coding System

20. Which of the following is a step in labeling a specimen?

    A) tying the requisition order to the specimen container

    B) placing the label on the body of the container, not the cap

    C) returning the sample to central processing to label

    D) having the patient inspect the specimen container

21. A patient who is about to have a lipid panel drawn mentions that they had a bagel on the way to the lab this morning. What should the phlebotomist do?

    A) proceed with the lab draw

    B) draw a discard tube before drawing the lipid panel

    C) alert the patient's provider to see if the patient's specimen should be rescheduled

    D) note that the patient is not fasting and proceed without any additional communication with the patient's provider

22. Blood specimens are transported in:

    A) biohazard bags

    B) a gloved hand

    C) any leakproof bag or box

    D) any of the above

23. The most common site of phlebotomy is the:

    A) popliteal fossa

    B) antecubital fossa

    C) axilla

    D) inguinal area

24. What does a breathalyzer machine test for?

   A) bacteria in the respiratory tract

   B) blood alcohol level

   C) blood in the mouth

   D) acid reflux

25. Which of the following is an acceptable IV site?

   A) a vein used for an IV 3 days ago

   B) bruised tissue

   C) burned hand tissue

   D) an arm with lymphedema

26. Which of the following veins is NOT found in the antecubital area?

   A) subclavian

   B) median cubital

   C) cephalic

   D) basilic

27. What is required for handling a preemployment drug screen?

   A) ensuring a legal transfer of the specimen

   B) outlining the tests that need to be conducted

   C) documenting the specimen's chain of custody

   D) assigning the testing to a specific employee

28. For patients with an M pattern in the antecubital fossa, what is the preferred vein for phlebotomy?

   A) median

   B) basilic

   C) cephalic

   D) median cubital

29. What is the term for the set amount a patient must pay out of pocket before their insurance company will pay for their care?

   A) coinsurance

   B) co-pay

   C) premium

   D) deductible

30. Gastric fluid is obtained from what part of the body?

   A) mouth

   B) stomach

   C) bladder

   D) colon

31. Which statement concerning informed consent is FALSE?

   A) Persons 17 years of age and younger may not give informed consent.

   B) A married minor may not give informed consent.

   C) A pregnant minor may give informed consent.

   D) An adult 18 years of age and older may give informed consent.

32. Which of the following sites is acceptable for a skin puncture for an adult?

   A) the antecubital fossa

   B) the back of the hand

   C) the pad of the index finger

   D) the pad of the ring finger

33. The maximum depth for an infant heel stick is:

   A) 1 mm

   B) 2 mm

   C) 1 cm

   D) 2 cm

34. Which of the following is NOT required for the transportation of specimens to an offsite laboratory?

A) a leakproof container stored on the floor of a vehicle

B) a vehicle that is used for transporting specimens only

C) protection for the specimens from heat and light

D) a specialized driver's license for transporting biological materials

35. Which of the following techniques is NOT recommended when performing a heel puncture for an infant?

A) puncturing the side of the heel

B) fanning or blowing on the skin to quicken drying after cleansing

C) positioning the infant's foot lower than its body

D) warming the heel first

36. Which of the following is TRUE about collecting an oral hormone specimen?

A) It needs to be collected within 30 minutes of waking up. Can be done @ home

B) It should be refrigerated or frozen if not processed within 24 hours.

C) It is frequently done for men with low albumin levels.

D) It is always done in a clinical setting.

37. A patient is having a panic attack and hyperventilating. How should the phlebotomist attempt to help this patient?

A) have the patient recount a positive childhood memory

B) give the patient a glass of water

C) tell the patient to take deep breaths

D) ask the patient to identify the source of their anxiety

38. When performing a heel stick on an infant, the first drop of blood should be:

A) collected in a microtube

B) placed in newborn screening paper

C) wiped away

D) stored in case additional blood is needed

39. Which of the following types of cells carries hemoglobin in the blood?

A) white blood cell

B) red blood cell

C) platelet

D) T cell

40. All of the following are reasons the phlebotomist should avoid aggressively squeezing the heel during an infant heel stick EXCEPT:

A) It can cause jaundice.

B) It is painful to the patient.

C) It can cause the cells to hemolyze.

D) It forces tissue fluid into the sample.

41. What is specific to how a stat specimen is processed?

A) It is processed at room temperature.

B) It can only be processed by certified laboratory personnel.

C) It is processed at the patient's bedside.

D) It is processed immediately, before any routine tests.

42. Which blood level is NOT elevated by hemolysis?

A) potassium

B) iron

C) ammonia

D) red blood cells

43. A patient rolls up their sleeve and presents their arm for a blood draw. This is an example of which type of consent?

A) informed consent

B) expressed consent

C) implied consent

D) indirect consent

44. Which of the following is <u>NOT a correct step</u> during a newborn screening?

A) touching the filter paper to the blood until the entire circle is filled

B) adding a second drop if the circle on the filter paper is incompletely filled

C) pressing the filter paper to the heel to fill the circle

D) laying the filter paper flat to dry

45. Which of the following types of blood has the highest oxygen level?

A) venous

B) arterial

C) clotted

D) hemolyzed

46. How is a light-sensitive sample stored for transport?

A) in black tubes

B) in a second specimen cup

C) in amber tubes

D) in a UV box

47. What disinfectant should be used to clean health care–related surfaces and equipment?

A) sodium hypochlorite

B) sodium hydroxide

C) diluted Lysol

D) 2:1 vinegar and distilled water solution

48. The procedure used to collect amniotic fluid is called:

A) an angioscopy

B) an amniotomy

C) an amniocentesis

D) a catheterization

49. When attempting phlebotomy on the arm, how far above the intended site of blood draw should the tourniquet be placed?

A) 0 – 1 inch

B) 2 – 4 inches

C) 5 – 7 inches

D) 7 – 10 inches

50. Why should the ends of the tourniquet be pointed away from the venipuncture site?

A) to prevent the tourniquet from coming loose

B) to occlude arterial flow

C) to prevent the veins from rolling

D) to avoid contaminating the skin at the blood draw site

51. Blood drawn from a fingertip is taken from which type of blood vessel?

A) vein

B) artery

C) arteriole

D) capillary

52. How long should a venipuncture site be allowed to air dry after being cleansed with an antiseptic?

A) 15 seconds

B) 30 seconds

C) 1 minute

D) 2 minutes

53. Which of the following minor patients is NOT able to give informed consent?

  A) a 12-year-old with a broken arm

  B) a 17-year-old seeking treatment for a sexually transmitted infection

  C) a pregnant minor

  D) an emancipated minor

54. Standard blood samples must be tested or centrifuged within:

  A) 1 hour

  B) 2 hours

  C) 4 hours

  D) 12 hours

55. What is a reason to reject a sample of cerebrospinal fluid?

  A) It was kept at room temperature.

  B) It contains clear fluid.

  C) It was collected over 24 hours ago.

  D) It is in a hematology tube.

56. What is the needle insertion angle for drawing blood from superficial hand veins?

  A) 10 degrees

  B) 20 degrees

  C) 45 degrees

  D) 90 degrees

57. A patient at a clinic becomes angry about the long wait to give a blood specimen. How should the phlebotomist react?

  A) attempt to restrain the patient

  B) speak loudly over the patient

  C) remain calm and use a normal voice

  D) call security

58. What is the phlebotomist's responsibility during bone marrow collection?

  A) perform a needlestick into the center of a large bone

  B) clean the area where the needle will be inserted

  C) mark the insertion site

  D) place the aspirated material onto a slide with a fixative

59. A blood sample is drawn into a purple-topped evacuated tube with EDTA. Which of the following could the sample be used for?

  A) basic metabolic panel

  B) potassium level

  C) complete blood count

  D) glucose

60. When during venipuncture should the tourniquet be removed?

  A) when the draw is complete

  B) before needle insertion

  C) once blood flow has been established

  D) after 10 seconds

61. What is the liquid part of blood called?

  A) serum

  B) saline

  C) plasma

  D) interstitial fluid

62. During venipuncture, the tourniquet should be tight enough to occlude _____ flow but not _____ flow.

  A) arterial; venous

  B) capillary; venous

  C) venous; arterial

  D) venous; capillary

63. A phlebotomist checks the refrigerator in which specimens are stored and finds that the temperature is 42°F (5.5°C). What is the first thing they should do? *35.6 – 50°F / 2 – 10°C*

   A) inform their supervisor

   B) move the specimens to another refrigerator

   C) label the tubes with the current temperature of the refrigerator

   D) No action is required.

64. The common cold, influenza, and HIV are caused by which type of infectious agent?

   A) bacteria

   B) protozoa

   C) virus

   D) helminth

65. The maximum amount of blood that can be safely drawn from a pediatric patient is primarily based on their:

   A) weight

   B) diet

   C) oxygen saturation

   D) pain tolerance

66. Where is serous fluid found?

   A) in the pericardial cavity

   B) in the subarachnoid space

   C) in bone marrow

   D) in the colon

67. The most common equipment used for pediatric phlebotomy is: *smallest & short*

   A) an 18-gauge syringe

   B) a 21-gauge ETS

   C) a 23-gauge syringe

   D) a 23-gauge butterfly

68. Why should the first evacuated tube drawn from a winged infusion system be discarded?

   A) Air in the tubing will cause the evacuated tube to underfill.

   B) Heparin in the tubing will contaminate the evacuated tube.

   C) The antiseptic used to clean the puncture site will contaminate the first tube.

   D) The flow of blood into the first tube hemolyzes the sample.

69. What is the difference between plasma and serum?

   A) Plasma contains clotting factors and serum does not.

   B) Plasma is collected by venipuncture and serum is collected by skin puncture.

   C) Plasma can be collected any time and serum is collected after fasting.

   D) Plasma has been centrifuged and serum has not been processed.

70. Contact with which of the following substances does NOT require the use of standard precautions?

   A) blood

   B) urine

   C) sweat

   D) vomit

71. Which of the following pediatric restraints is NOT age appropriate?

   A) a 1-month-old swaddled with one arm out of the blanket

   B) a 2-year-old sitting in a chair, with the parent in the room

   C) a 4-year-old in the parent's lap, facing the parent in a bear hug

   D) a 14-year-old sitting in a phlebotomy chair with the parent present

72. Which of the following is a sign that a sample has been hemolyzed?

A) The tube is cracked.

B) The sample has casts in it.

C) The stopper on the tube is loose.

D) The serum is pink after centrifugation.

73. What test is used to diagnose a *Helicobacter pylori* infection? *Causes stomach ulcer direct contact through saliva, vomit or stool food or water*

A) breathalyzer

B) C-urea breath test

C) lumbar puncture

D) sputum culture

74. A topical anesthetic can be applied prior to venipuncture beginning at what age?

A) 1 month

B) 6 months

C) 12 months

D) 24 months

75. Which of the following is an example of transmission of an infectious agent through direct contact? *physical*

A) kissing an infected person

B) inhaling droplets from the sneeze of an infected person

C) standing near an infected person who is coughing

D) eating contaminated food

76. When should therapeutic drug monitoring trough levels be collected?

A) immediately before the drug is administered

B) immediately after the drug is administered

C) 1 hour after the drug is administered

D) 2 hours after the drug is administered

77. Platelets are essential for:

A) fighting infection

B) oxygen delivery

C) destroying pathogens

D) coagulation

78. What is the first step for a patient to take when collecting a clean-catch urine sample?

A) wash their hands *drugs clean hands*

B) void the first half of the urine into the toilet

C) put on gloves

D) clean the urinary meatus

79. Geriatric vascular changes result in all of the following EXCEPT:

A) decreased risk of hypertension

B) loss of elasticity of vessels

C) decreased blood flow from impaired peripheral circulation

D) narrowing of blood vessels

80. Under CLIA, what is the term for simple laboratory tests with a low risk for incorrect results that may be performed by anyone who follows the manufacturer's directions?

A) elementary tests

B) moderate-complexity tests

C) high-complexity tests

D) waived tests

81. A phlebotomist is questioning a patient through an interpreter. Who should questions be directed to?

A) the interpreter

B) the physician

C) the patient's family

D) the patient

82. A person with blood type O has which of the following plasma antibodies?

   A) anti-A

   B) anti-B

   C) neither anti-A nor anti-B

   D) both anti-A and anti-B

83. When performing phlebotomy on a patient with dementia, which of the following is NOT appropriate behavior by the phlebotomist?

   A) talking quickly through their introduction to the patient

   B) allowing extra time for the patient to respond

   C) using simple, short statements

   D) being calm and understanding if the patient is agitated or confused

84. What color is the top of tubes used for blood bank specimens?

   A) pink

   B) red

   C) royal blue

   D) green

85. Rh immune globulin (brand name RhoGAM) is given to pregnant people who are Rh negative to prevent which of the following serious problems for the infant?

   A) congenital heart defects

   B) infection

   C) hemolytic disease of the newborn

   D) seizures

86. A dipstick can be used in urinalysis to test for all of the following EXCEPT:

   A) pH level

   B) red blood cells

   C) parasites

   D) glucose

87. Which type of waste is NOT matched with its correct disposal container?

   A) capillary tubes: sharps container

   B) feces: toilet

   C) gauze with small amount of blood: regular garbage can

   D) linen heavily soiled by blood: dirty linen receptacle

88. What is included in the comprehensive metabolic panel (CMP) that is NOT included in the basic metabolic panel (BMP)?

   A) electrolyte level tests

   B) glucose level tests

   C) liver function tests

   D) kidney function tests

89. Prothrombin time (PT) is used to assess:

   A) coagulation

   B) liver function

   C) kidney function

   D) electrolyte levels

90. Which precaution must a phlebotomist take when checking the blood pressure of an HIV-positive patient?

   A) wearing gloves

   B) wearing a gown

   C) using contact precautions

   D) washing hands

91. A crossmatch test checks for:

   A) the presence of bacteria in the blood

   B) the type of antibiotics that will treat a patient's infection

   C) the compatibility of donor blood with recipient blood

   D) the average blood glucose level over the past 3 months

92. Which of the following types of urine specimens is used specifically for diabetic screening?

A) random

B) clean-catch midstream

C) 2-hour postprandial

D) 24-hour

93. Which of the following blood tests checks for the average size of red blood cells?

A) erythrocyte count

B) mean corpuscular hemoglobin (MCH)

C) hematocrit

D) mean corpuscular volume (MCV)

94. A localized dilation or bulging in the wall of a blood vessel is also known as:

A) an embolism

B) a hemorrhoid

C) an aneurysm

D) a blood clot

95. The phlebotomist has finished drawing blood and notes that the sharps container is full. What should they do?

A) Exchange the full container for a new one.

B) Place the syringe on top of the container so it will not roll off.

C) Push the syringe into the container as well as it will fit.

D) Put the syringe in their pocket and dispose of it in another room.

96. Which of the following tests is NOT elevated with inflammation?

A) white blood cell count (WBC)

B) C-reactive protein (CRP)

C) international normalized ratio (INR)

D) erythrocyte sedimentation rate (ESR)

97. Which of the following should a patient NOT do before a sputum culture?

A) use antibacterial mouthwash

B) use antibacterial hand soap

C) wear restrictive clothing

D) take an antihistamine

98. Pregnancy can be confirmed by testing for:

A) human chorionic gonadotropin (HCG)

B) thyroid stimulating hormone (TSH)

C) C-reactive protein (CRP)

D) cold agglutinins

99. Which of the following statements is correct in terms of the order in which to put on or remove PPE?

A) When removing PPE, gloves are removed last.

B) When removing PPE, the mask is removed before the gown.

C) When putting on PPE, gloves are put on before the mask.

D) When putting on PPE, the gown is put on last.

100. A risk of drawing blood from the median cubital vein is possible damage to the:

A) radial artery

B) brachial artery

C) lateral cutaneous nerve

D) median nerve

ANSWER KEY

1. **B)** **Correct.** The SA node starts the electrical conduction pathway for the heart by producing a regular impulse that causes the atria to contract. On an EKG this is reflected by the P wave.

2. **C)** **Correct.** An introduction should include a greeting, the phlebotomist's name and title, and the reason they are visiting the patient.

3. **D)** **Correct.** Casts are cylindrical structures in urine. They may contain red blood cells, white blood cells, or fats and can indicate kidney disease.

4. **B)** **Correct.** At least 2 identifiers are required to confirm a patient's identity.

5. **C)** **Correct.** Speaking in short, simple sentences while remaining calm will help de-escalate the patient's mood.

6. **D)** **Correct.** The patient's room number should not be used to confirm a patient's identity.

7. **B)** **Correct.** The pulmonary artery carries this blood away from the right side of the heart into the lungs to be oxygenated. It is the only artery that carries deoxygenated blood.

8. **C)** **Correct.** A temporary name and number will be assigned to an unconscious patient. This will be cross-referenced with a permanent number once their identity is confirmed. Use the assigned temporary name and number for ID confirmation until then.

9. **A)** **Correct.** A lab requisition is considered a legal document and is part of the patient's medical record.

10. **C)** **Correct.** Proper confirmation of a patient's identity is the most important step in specimen collection. The phlebotomist should not proceed until any discrepancies have been addressed.

11. **A)** **Correct.** Patients who are unconscious, mentally impaired, or minors require additional steps to verify their identity, such as confirmation from the provider, nurse, parent, or legal guardian.

12. **C)** **Correct.** Capillaries are the site of gas exchange. Oxygenated blood flows from the arterioles to the capillaries, and deoxygenated blood moves from the capillaries to the venules.

13. **A)** **Correct.** Other symptoms of shock include difficulty breathing, decreased urine output, and a rapid pulse.

14. **D)** **Correct.** Postprandial means "after a meal."

15. **A)** **Correct.** Test collection priority is stat, ASAP (or pre-op/post-op), timed, fasting, and routine.

16. **B)** **Correct.** The ordered test is given a number to track its components through collecting and processing.

17. **A)** **Correct.** The basal state is the body's metabolic state after a patient has been fasting for 12 hours.

18. **C)** **Correct.** The use of a urinary collection bag decreases the high risk of infection from using a catheter.

19. **B)** **Correct.** Current Procedural Terminology (CPT) codes use a standardized set of five-digit codes to identify medical, surgical, or diagnostic services.

20. **B)** **Correct.** The label for a specimen must stay on the container it is held in.

21. **C)** **Correct.** If the patient has not met the testing requirements (fasting is required for a lipid panel), the phlebotomist should contact the patient's provider before proceeding. If the provider approves the test to be run anyway, make a note in the chart that the patient did

not fast and that the test was approved by the provider.

22. **A)** **Correct.** Lab specimens must be transported in a leakproof bag labeled as biohazard.

23. **B.** **Correct.** The antecubital fossa is the depression on the inside of the elbow.

24. **B)** **Correct.** A breathalyzer is a device that analyzes the breath for the presence of alcohol.

25. **A)** **Correct.** Do not draw blood from an IV site if it was used for an IV less than 2 days ago.

26. **A)** **Correct.** The subclavian vein is located more proximally, near the clavicle.

27. **C)** **Correct.** Chain of custody is the procedure for handling pre-employment drug screens.

28. **A)** **Correct.** For patients with M-patterned veins, the median vein is the preferred choice. The median cephalic vein can also be considered.

29. **D)** **Correct.** The patient's deductible is the set amount a patient is responsible for paying before the insurance company will pay for care.

30. **B)** **Correct.** The overproduction or underproduction of stomach acid, the presence of an ulcer or bile, and the effectiveness of anti-ulcer medication are some of the issues that are diagnosed with a gastric fluid sample.

31. **B)** **Correct.** In general, minors may not give informed consent, but exceptions include married and pregnant minors.

32. **D)** **Correct.** In adults, the medial or lateral side of the pad of the middle or ring finger is an acceptable skin puncture site.

33. **B)** **Correct.** The maximum depth of skin puncture for an infant heel stick is 2 mm.

34. **D)** **Correct.** Drivers transporting specimens to offsite laboratories do not require specialized licenses.

35. **B)** **Correct.** Do not blow on, fan, or pat the skin to quicken drying after cleansing.

36. **A)** **Correct.** Oral hormone tests can be done at home because specimens need to be collected within 30 minutes of waking up and may need to be repeated throughout the day.

37. **C)** **Correct.** Taking slow, deep breaths can change the patient's physiological response to the panic attack and possibly alleviate it.

38. **C)** **Correct.** The first drop of blood from a skin puncture should be wiped away to prevent contamination from tissue fluid or antiseptic residue.

39. **B)** **Correct.** Red blood cells contain hemoglobin, which has an iron component that transports oxygen. It also makes the red blood cells appear red in color.

40. **A)** **Correct.** Squeezing the heel during a heel stick can cause cell hemolysis, be painful to the patient and can force tissue fluid into the sample. Jaundice occurs when high bilirubin levels cause skin to appear yellow in color.

41. **D)** **Correct.** The health care provider is notified of the results of a stat specimen as soon as they are ready.

42. **D)** **Correct.** Red blood cell levels decrease during hemolysis because they are broken apart.

43. **C)** **Correct.** When a patient rolls up their sleeve and offers their arm for a blood draw, this is an example of implied consent.

44. **B)** **Correct.** Only one drop of blood can be used to fill each circle on newborn screening filter paper. Using more than one drop per circle can cause blood layering and false results.

45. B) Correct. Arterial blood is richest in oxygen. It has left the heart and is bringing oxygen to the tissues and organs.

46. C) Correct. Amber tubes are used for light-sensitive specimens such as bilirubin. The tube may be wrapped in aluminum foil as well.

47. A) Correct. Sodium hypochlorite is commonly known as bleach.

48. C) Correct. During an amniocentesis a doctor uses ultrasound to guide a needle into a pregnant patient's abdomen to collect a sample of amniotic fluid.

49. B) Correct. The tourniquet should be placed 2 – 4 inches (5 – 10 cm) above the intended blood draw site.

50. D) Correct. The ends of the tourniquet should be pointed away from the venipuncture site to prevent contamination.

51. D) Correct. Capillaries are the smallest of the blood vessels. They connect the arterial and venous systems. They are found near the surface of the skin and are often used for collection of a blood glucose check or for newborn screening tests.

52. B) Correct. The site should air dry for 30 seconds after skin has been cleansed.

53. A) Correct. Minors can give informed consent in certain circumstances. Otherwise, consent must be given by the patient's guardian.

54. B) Correct. Standard blood samples should be tested within 2 hours. The samples should be separated via centrifugation if processing will take longer than 2 hours.

55. C) Correct. Cerebrospinal fluid samples need to be transported immediately at room temperature for testing.

56. A) Correct. Superficial hand veins need a shallow insertion angle, about 10 degrees.

57. C) Correct. Remaining calm and speaking in a normal tone and volume can help calm the patient down.

58. D) Correct. Bone marrow aspiration is an invasive test performed by a doctor. It involves suctioning bone marrow from the center of a long bone with a large needle.

59. C) Correct. Lavender- or purple-topped tubes contain the anticoagulant EDTA, which keeps the cells for a complete blood count from clotting.

60. C) Correct. Once blood flow has been established, the tourniquet should be released.

61. C) Correct. Plasma is the clear yellow fluid part of the blood. Electrolyte, fats, clotting factors, blood cells (red and white), and platelets are suspended in the plasma.

62. C) Correct. The tourniquet should be tight enough to occlude venous flow (to make veins more prominent and easier to see/locate) but not occlude arterial flow.

63. D) Correct. An appropriate temperature for a refrigerator that is used for storing specimens is between 35.6°F and 50°F (2°C and 10°C).

64. C) Correct. Viruses are responsible for the common cold, influenza, and HIV (human immunodeficiency virus).

65. A) Correct. A patient's weight determines the maximum amount of blood that can be safely drawn. The maximum draw in mL is about twice a patient's weight in kilograms (e.g., a patient who weighs 10 kg has a max draw of 20 mL).

66. A) Correct. Serous fluid is also found in the peritoneal cavity and the pleural cavity.

67. D) Correct. A 23-gauge butterfly needle is usually used for pediatric patients.

68. A) Correct. Underfilling an evacuated tube can affect the necessary blood volume or the additive-to-blood ratio. The first tube should be discarded after collection to prevent erroneous results.

69. **A)** **Correct.** When the clotting factors (fibrinogen) are removed from plasma, the serum is what is left. After blood is collected and allowed to clot, it is placed in the centrifuge. The spinning in the centrifuge will separate the blood into 2 layers: serum and clotted blood. This is usually done in a serum separator tube (SST).

70. **C)** **Correct.** Standard precautions are recommended whenever the phlebotomist comes in contact with blood or body fluids that could transmit blood-borne pathogens. Sweat does not require standard precautions.

71. **B)** **Correct.** Toddlers and young children should be positioned in a parent's lap in a bear hug or back to chest position.

72. **D)** **Correct.** Hemolysis is the breaking apart of the red blood cells. It makes the serum look pink.

73. **B)** **Correct.** *Helicobacter pylori* is a bacterium that can cause stomach ulcers.

74. **C)** **Correct.** A topical anesthetic may be used in children older than 12 months.

75. **A)** **Correct.** Direct contact is the transmission of infectious agents through physical contact between two people, such as kissing.

76. **A)** **Correct.** Trough levels are collected when drug serum levels should be the lowest, immediately before the next dose is scheduled.

77. **D)** **Correct.** Platelets play a key role in blood clotting. They are the first cells to respond to an injury.

78. **A)** **Correct.** Patients should wash their hands.

79. **A)** **Correct.** Geriatric vascular changes include narrowing of blood vessels, decreased blood flow because their circulation is impaired, and loss of vessel elasticity (increases risk of vein collapse).

80. **D)** **Correct.** CLIA waived tests do not require quality assurance protocols because they are easy to perform and have a low risk of erroneous results.

81. **D)** **Correct.** Medical professionals should always speak directly to their patient when the patient has an interpreter, regardless of whether the patient can hear or speak English.

82. **D)** **Correct.** Type O blood type has anti-A and anti-B plasma antibodies (agglutinins).

83. **A)** **Correct.** Talk slowly to patients who have dementia and allow them extra time to respond.

84. **A)** **Correct.** Blood bank specimens are collected in tubes with pink or lavender tops.

85. **C)** **Correct.** The "negative" or "positive" listed after a blood type indicates the Rh factor. An Rh-negative pregnant patient may make antibodies against the Rh-positive red blood cells in the fetus. If this happens, the fetus's blood cells will burst or hemolyze, causing severe, sometimes fatal anemia.

86. **C)** **Correct.** A dipstick placed into a urine sample tests for pH, red blood cells, and glucose. The microscopic portion of the urinalysis may be helpful in identifying bacteria, blood cells, parasites, and tumor cells.

87. **D)** **Correct.** Linen that is lightly soiled can go in the dirty linen receptacle; however, linen that is heavily soiled by blood should be placed in a biohazard bag.

88. **C)** **Correct.** A BMP includes kidney function (BUN, Cr), glucose, and electrolytes (Na, K, Cl, CO_3). A CMP is all the BMP tests plus liver function tests (AST, ALT), bilirubin, and proteins (albumin).

89. A) **Correct.** PT is used to determine how long it takes for a patient's blood to clot. It is drawn in patients who are on warfarin (Coumadin).

90. D) **Correct.** Hand washing is sufficient since taking a client's blood pressure does not involve contact with blood or secretions.

91. C) **Correct.** A crossmatch test checks to make sure that donor blood will not cause a reaction with the patient's blood. Incompatible blood can have dangerous consequences for the recipient.

92. C) **Correct.** Urine is collected 2 hours after a meal to test for glycosuria, or glucose in the urine.

93. D) **Correct.** MCV measures the average size of red blood cells.

94. C) **Correct.** An aneurysm is caused by a weakening of the blood vessel wall.

95. A) **Correct.** The full container should be replaced with a new one.

96. C) **Correct.** INR is used to measure the effectiveness of the blood thinner warfarin (Coumadin) and is not correlated with inflammation.

97. A) **Correct.** Using an antibacterial mouthwash before a sputum specimen collection can cause an inaccurate result.

98. A) **Correct.** HCG levels increase during pregnancy.

99. B) **Correct.** When removing PPE, gloves are removed first, then eye protection, mask, and gown. Hand hygiene is performed last. When putting on PPE, hand hygiene is first, followed by gown, mask, eye protection, and finally, gloves.

100. B) **Correct.** The median cubital vein overlies the brachial artery.

Follow the link below to access your second NHA Phlebotomy practice test:

www.ascenciatestprep.com/nha-phlebotomy-online-resources

Made in the USA
Las Vegas, NV
11 March 2023